Medicinal Herb Gardening

10 Plants for the Self-Reliant Homestead Prepper

I0456186

Jill b.

ISBN: 1530603161
ISBN-13: 978-1530603169

CONTENTS

1 INTRODUCTION

Statements in this book have not been evaluated by the Food and Drug Administration. Information in this book is not intended to diagnose, treat, cure or prevent any disease.

In the US, where big pharma rules, natural remedies are often brushed off as quackery. While modern medicine has a place in our society, in a grid-down or rural homestead situation, having a medicinal garden in your backyard may mean the difference between life and death.

I am an accidental homesteader. Facing grid-down situations are a part of life in the Colorado foothills. Fortunately, we were never faced with a life and death situation. Living in that environment taught us the importance of being prepared and self-sufficiency. In the first book of the SHTF Series, "Foraging: A Beginner's Guide to Wild Edible and Medicinal Plants" (http://byjillb.com), I covered important beneficial "weeds" that grow in most of the US. I will therefore not include useful plants like dandelion, cattail and plantain in this book.

Instead, I'd like to take our homesteading or survival prepping to the next level - planting, cultivating and harvesting medicinal herbs and foods that are not as easy to forage in the wild.

Since there is an abundance of healing and medicinal plants in Nature, it would be impossible for me to include them all in this book. Instead, given the struggles I experienced trying to grow in a short-season, high-altitude climate, I have narrowed the list of plants down to useful medicinal plants that are easy to grow in most of the lower 48 states. The ten plants I curated were carefully chosen for their multi-purposes. All are not only medicinal but also edible. Many have additional utilitarian uses.

I have written this book with the beginning homesteader, gardener and/or survival prepper in mind. This book, however, assumes basic gardening knowledge which I covered in "The Modern American Frugal Housewife Book #2 - Organic Gardening" (http://byjillb.com).

Let food be thy medicine and medicine be thy food -
Hippocrates

2 CAYENNE

Native to Central and South America, Cayenne is named after the city of Cayenne in French Guiana. Cayenne pepper (*Capsicum annuum*) is part of the Solanaceae family, also known as the Nightshade family. This family includes tomatoes, potatoes, eggplants, as well as deadly nightshades like tobacco.

Cayenne is a perennial in tropical and subtropical climates. They are normally grown as annual plants in temperate climates but can be overwintered indoors. There are many varieties of cayenne peppers which vary in appearance, with their shrubby plants ranging in heights from two to six feet. Its fruit are red, long and ovate, with a long row of small, flat seeds within.

The edible fruits are spicy and pungent, with a rating of between 30,000 to 50,000 Scoville units. The fruits are commonly used fresh, dried or preserved in vinegar. It is often used in a variety of Asian cuisines and is often used as an ingredient in hot sauces. What is less known though, is Cayenne pepper's medicinal qualities.

Uses

Healing Agent

Native Americans have used Cayenne as food and medicine for thousands of years before it was later introduced to

Chinese and Ayurvedic medicine to treat various ailments including frostbite and myalgia.

Cayenne seems to have excellent regenerative properties, especially on the heart. According to a medical study, live heart tissue placed in distilled water and fed nothing but Cayenne pepper, continued to grow and produce tissue. Although it had no control glands, the heart tissue grew continually and stayed alive for 17 years until it was destroyed for analysis.

The late herbalist and medical doctor, Dr. Christopher, and Dr. Nowell, Dr. Christopher's teacher at the Herbal College in Canada, attributed the healing of ulcers, heart attacks, asthma, arthritis, the hardening of arteries and other ailments suffered by both their patients and Dr. Christopher himself, to Cayenne. By living a healthy lifestyle and diet, and taking a teaspoon of Cayenne three times a day, Dr. Christopher was able to heal his high blood pressure. Adding Cayenne to your food may also be used to help to keep your body temperature up in cold temperatures.

According to Dr. Christopher, a few droppers full (1 dropper is approximately 35 drops or 1/4 teaspoon or 1 ml) of Cayenne tincture or a cup of Cayenne tea, which consists of a teaspoon of Cayenne in a cup of hot water may help during or to prevent a heart attack. If a heart attack is in progress or had already happened, Dr. Christopher suggested administering a teaspoon of extract, or a teaspoon of Cayenne in a glass of hot water every 15 minutes until the crisis has passed.

Tinctures are basically herbs infused in a liquid solvent such as vinegar, consumable alcohol, honey or vegetable glycerin.

Of these, apple cider vinegar, food grade vegetable glycerin or 100 proof alcohol (50% alcohol and 50% water) are some of the more common solvents used. If you use a lower proof alcohol, you will need to let your infusion sit for longer periods of time before use. A lower proof alcohol tincture will also not last as long as a high proof one can.

In my opinion, apple cider vinegar is a lesser choice when making most tinctures because they tend to not last as long. Food grade vegetable glycerin is a decent choice for making tinctures especially for children's remedies because of its sweet taste. You can find food grade vegetable glycerin on Amazon. In large quantities, Essential Depot (http://bit.ly/1v7V3rE)* sells it at a reasonable price. However, in the case of Cayenne extract, using 100% proof alcohol is a better choice as it is one of the best preservatives that can extract Cayenne's beneficial components.

Cayenne Extract Tincture

To make your Cayenne extract, stuff a clean, dry wide-mouthed jar full of peppers. You can also fill the jar halfway with Cayenne powder. If you are using dried peppers or pepper powder, make sure that they are at least 40,000 Scoville heat units (this includes Cayenne, Tabasco and Aji peppers). Pour the alcohol up to the neck of the jar, making sure that the peppers are completely covered in alcohol.

Screw the lid on tightly and shake the jar gently. Store the jar in a dark, cool place for at least a month. The longer the tincture is allowed to sit, the better. After at least a month, wear rubber gloves and strain the tincture through a clean cheesecloth, squeezing out as much tincture as you can. It's best to store your finished tincture in amber glass dropper bottles.

Wound Healing Agent

According to Dr. Christopher, Cayenne is one of the best natural remedies for cuts. He notes, "...*cayenne is a counter-irritant. Cayenne brings the blood to the surface to take away any toxic poisons and start[s] the healing. The redness comes to the skin from the blood that has rushed to the surface to assist carrying off wastes.*" Additionally, a 2003 study published by Medical Mycology proved that Cayenne pepper has anti-fungal and antibacterial properties, which can help to disinfect wounds.

Dr. Christopher further notes that Cayenne powder, when dumped on deep cuts and wounds, including gunshot wounds, has helped to stop the bleeding. To prevent shock, Master Herbalist, David Christopher suggests drinking at least a tablespoon of Cayenne pepper mixed in hot water.

The reason for Cayenne pepper's effectiveness is because Cayenne reacts in the body and equalizes the blood pressure. The circulatory system is a closed pressure system. When the body suffers a cut or open wound, the pressure balance is disrupted. Cayenne equalizes the pressure, which slows the blood flowing out of the wound. This process allows the blood to clot more quickly. When Cayenne is applied externally and directly onto the wound, the clotting occurs even faster.

Natural Pesticide

In addition to its medicinal benefits, Cayenne can also be used as a natural pesticide and animal deterrent. According to "Rodale's Ultimate Encyclopedia of Organic Gardening", hot peppers repel pests like aphids, cabbage maggots and spider mites. Hot pepper sprays work best against flying insects that feed on flowers, fruits and leaves.

Cayenne Pepper Spray

To make a Cayenne spray, briefly blend 1/2 cup of Cayenne peppers and a few optional cloves of peeled garlic with 2 cups of water. Strain the solids from the liquid. Use a spray bottle to apply the Cayenne liquid.

You can also dust Cayenne powder around the base of the stem of plants to deter crawling pests like cutworms or cabbage maggots. It may also repel larger garden pests like raccoons, rabbits and deer.

Even though Cayenne does not pose a threat to the environment like other chemical pesticides might, it is important to note that using Cayenne as a pesticide may also be toxic to beneficial bugs like bees. Also make sure that you do not apply the spray against the wind as it may cause nasal, lung or skin irritation.

Weapon

In addition to using Cayenne against intrusive bugs and animals, you can also use it against humans. It is used in Asia as a weapon and is a common non-lethal, self-defense option. Since it is a renewable resource, you can use it in situations where you want to conserve ammunition or where firearms are not needed. It may be an especially useful weapon during a societal or economic collapse. Remember that there is a risk of injury when making and using pepper spray

Caution: Wear gloves and safety eye goggles and prepare your pepper spray in a well ventilated area.

Cayenne peppers at the lower Scoville Heat Unit (SHU) range of 30,000 to 60,000 SHU is suitable for this use. However, you may also opt to use more potent peppers like Habaneros (350,000-650,000 SHU), or Ghost Peppers or Naga Jolokia Peppers (800,000 - 1,500,000 SHU) which are considered some of the hottest peppers in the world.

While you can use water as the liquid carrier for your spray, using an Isopropyl rubbing alcohol, vinegar or oil spray (use mineral or baby oil) will keep longer than a water carrier spray which will last for about 2 weeks. As an added advantage over using water as a carrier, Isopropyl rubbing alcohol and vinegar are irritants while using mineral or baby oil as a carrier will make the spray adhere more to skin and clothes.

You can use 1-2 ounce spray bottles that are available at most store toiletries sections. You can also use larger 24-32 oz spray bottles which you can find at the Dollar Store or Walmart. You can also make a much larger spray dispenser using 1-4 gallon garden hand pump pressure sprayer which is normally used for weed or pest control. These sprayers can usually be found at home improvement stores or feed stores

Naturally, you will need more peppers to make larger containers of spray solution. Also, the larger the spray container, the less control you tend to have over the mist so make sure to practice extreme caution when using the spray. Test your container by filling it with water to make sure that the container you use does not leak when laid on its side, when tilted or after use. Do not use a container that may spill or leak spray solution where you do not want it to.

Cayenne Pepper Spray

This recipe yields about one pint of pepper spray. Use rubber gloves, safety eye goggles and a face mask or respirator, especially if you are sensitive.

Ingredients

1. At least 6 dried Cayenne (or hotter) peppers or 8 Tbsp Cayenne powder.
2. 1 large or 2 medium-sized garlic bulbs or 2 tablespoons of garlic powder.
3. 1 tablespoon of ground black pepper (optional but helps to cause coughing).
4. 2 Tbsp baby or mineral oil.
5. 12 oz of white vinegar or Isopropyl rubbing alcohol.

Method

1. Grind the peppers and garlic in a blender or chop is as finely as you can and place it in a bowl.
2. Add the baby or mineral oil and blend/mix.
3. Gradually add the vinegar or alcohol into the mixture.
4. Let the mixture sit covered overnight in a cool place.
5. Using a strainer or cheesecloth, strain the mixture carefully into a storage container or into your spray bottle.
6. If you used mineral oil, discard the remaining solids. Otherwise, you can compost it.
7. Store your spray in a cool dry place or in the fridge.

An alcohol/vinegar mixture should last 1-3 months.

Note: Use soap and hot water to clean out the blender and other cooking utensils. If you used mineral oil, you can clean it out using a solution of bleach and water. Remember to keep your gloves and safety goggles on when you are cleaning up.

Food

Finally, most people are familiar with using Cayenne pepper as a food spice. Use it fresh, dried, powdered or preserved to give your dishes a different flavor or dimension. It will also come in handy in providing flavor in grid-down situations when access to many ingredients may be limited.

What is less known is that young Cayenne pepper leaves are edible when cooked (not raw). In parts of Asia, they are normally prepared as a green vegetable, or added to soups or stews. However, always practice caution when consuming a new food because some people may exhibit allergies to certain foods.

Cultivation

Cayenne is generally a perennial in tropical and subtropical regions. It is grown as an annual in temperate climates but can be overwintered if it is protected from frost or moved indoors. Peppers prefer to grow in warm temperatures and in moist, nutrient-rich soil. The plants grow between 2-3 feet in height. Plants should be spaced 1-3 feet apart. The plants may be planted more closely but the yields of each plant will diminish.

Peppers grow easily from seed, which is generally the cheapest way to cultivate Cayenne. However, the plant takes about 100 days to mature from seed. In areas with a long growing season, you can sow seeds directly outdoors 10-14 days before the last frost date.

In colder climates, you can start seeds indoors about 2 months before the last frost date. The seedlings should be kept in an area that has at least 5 hours of sunlight but a location that receives 12 hours of sunlight is ideal.

The seeds should be planted in individual pots as the plants do not like to be transplanted. Use a light planting medium that has good drainage. The soil needs to be kept moist but not wet and the temperature should be maintained at 75°F. You can use a transparent plastic dome to help keep the plant environment more constant. The seeds will sprout in about 16-20 days.

When the seedlings reach about 4-6 inches tall, start hardening them off by taking them outside to a shaded area and bringing them back indoors in the evening or when the weather gets bad. Gradually expose them to more elements over a week of hardening off. Only save the seedlings that have dark leaves and strong stems. Choose the same if you are buying your transplants. Resist the urge to buy plants that are already fruiting because contrary to their attractiveness, these plants will not produce well.

Transplant the seedlings outdoors only after the outside soil temperature is at least 60°F. You usually have to wait about 3 weeks after the last frost for the soil temperatures to reach this temperature. Choose a cloudy day or provide some temporary shade when you transplant your peppers to reduce shock.

If your planting location is not sheltered from the wind, have supports already in place before transplanting. Adding your supports after transplanting can damage the plant roots. Secure your plants to the support loosely with cloth strips. You can also deter pests like cutworms by placing a cardboard collar around each plant. The collar should be pushed into the ground at least 1" deep. Emptied toilet paper cardboard rolls are good this purpose. Be prepared to protect your plants from cold or rain with cleaned, emptied plastic milk jugs.

Water your pepper plants evenly and well. Mulch deeply around the plants with light mulch like straw to help to retain moisture and to keep the weeds out. Make sure that your plants do not suffer from dry spells as the lack of water can cause the peppers to turn bitter. Provide the plants with shade if temperatures exceed 90°F. High temperatures can make the plants wilt or cause the flowers to fall off. Unless you notice slow growth or pale leaves, peppers in general do not need to be fertilized. If needed, apply compost tea or fish emulsion to your plants.

Harvesting

Harvest your peppers before they ripen and mature to encourage the plant to continue fruiting. The plant may stop production if you leave mature fruit on it. Mature fruit have the fullest flavor but only leave the fruit to mature and ripen when the season is over. Peppers usually turn red when ripe but colors can vary from purple to black to brown to ivory depending on the variety.

Never pull the peppers off the plant. Use a sharp, clean knife to cut them off instead. Frost will damage the fruit so pick all the fruit before any expected frost. If you have hot peppers that underwent a light (not hard) frost, you can save them by turning them into hot sauce.

Allow unripe peppers to ripen in a cool, dry place indoors. You can also pull the plants up by the roots and hang them to dry, allowing the fruits to ripen that way. Fruit preservation techniques include drying (hot) peppers, freezing (without blanching) and by preserving (hot) peppers in distilled white vinegar.

Propagation

Harvest seeds only from fully ripe peppers. Saving pepper seeds is easy - cut off the bottom of the fruit and carefully remove the seeds from the core. If you have a large number of seeds to process, separate your good seeds from the immature ones by allowing the mature seeds to sink to the bottom of a container of water.

Drain off any debris and immature seeds that float to the top. The seeds usually do not need additional cleaning. Spread the seeds on non-glossy newspaper in a cool location to dry. The seeds are dry enough to be stored if they break when folded.

3 COMFREY

Comfrey (*Symphytum officinale* L.) is a perennial plant which is part of the Boraginaceae or Borage family of plants. A European native, its green, upright stem can easily grow up to 5 feet tall and bears large, hairy leaves that are fairly broad. Comfrey bears groups of small, pretty bell-shaped flowers which range in color from cream to pink to purple. It prefers growing in damp, grassy areas like on river banks.

Comfrey is also known as boneset, knitbone, gum plant, slippery root, bruise-wort, wound wort or healing herb. Its common names hint at the healing power of this very useful plant.

Uses

Healing Agent

As some of its common names suggest, Comfrey, when used as an herb, has been used historically as a healing agent to help heal wounds and ulcers, as well so to mend or "knit" bones, flesh and sinew. Comfrey has been used by the Ancients -- from the Greeks to the Turks to stop bleeding and to heal battle wounds.

As an experiment, we applied a Comfrey poultice on my husband's hunting wound. The section which the poultice was applied healed considerably faster than the area that was not exposed to Comfrey. In another incident, my skeptical mother applied a Comfrey infusion on a skin condition that medical doctors told her was incurable. After applying the Comfrey for about 2 weeks, her condition cleared.

Scientifically, allantoin is credited for Comfrey's healing prowess. It is believed that Comfrey produces allantoin so that it can grow and heal itself quickly. Its roots contain twice as much allantoin as the leaves do. Allantoin, when absorbed by the skin helps to rejuvenate and multiply healthy cells. According to Dr. Christopher, Comfrey does not help to multiply malignant cells. In his book, he notes that in his 40 years of medical practice (before herbal medical practice was outlawed in the US), he had successfully used Comfrey for asthma, bruises, cuts burns and many types of wounds.

Because Comfrey can help to heal wounds so fast, it is very important to make sure that all wounds are thoroughly cleaned out before applying Comfrey. Otherwise, dirt particles or foreign substances may get embedded in the healing process. Do not use Comfrey on deep puncture wounds as the deep wound may not heal fast enough to keep up with the speed of healing on the skin surface. Many sources also caution against applying Comfrey on open wounds because of the risk of Comfrey causing liver damage.

The presence of toxic alkaloids makes Comfrey a controlled herb in many countries including the US. However, in a grid-down or dire situation, having Comfrey in your medicinal arsenal might come in very helpful.

Comfrey Poultice

Using Comfrey in external applications is believed to be generally safe. Do not apply fresh Comfrey leaves directly on the wound because the hairs on the leaves can be extremely irritating on the skin. Instead, chop a few Comfrey leaves up then place the leaves in a clean bowl. Pour hot (but not boiling) water over them. Allow the water to cool (save the water for watering your plants).

Once cooled, remove the leaves and squeeze out the excess water. The mash can now be applied on the skin. Use young leaves where possible for this purpose. Place the poultice on the affected area and use a cloth or bandage to hold the poultice in place.

Comfrey Burn Paste

You can also make a Comfrey burn paste using Dr. Christopher's formula of mixing equal parts of Comfrey leaf or powder, wheat germ oil and honey. Use raw, organic honey where possible. Apply the paste directly to the burn or wound and allow it to absorb into the skin. Apply more when the paste is absorbed. There is no need to remove the earlier application before applying more.

Fertilizer

Comfrey has a deep tap root that can grow several feet below the ground, drawing important nutrients from the subsoil into itself. Comfrey is high in nitrogen (N), potassium (K) and phosphorus (P), the three most essential nutrients for plant growth. According to a study in British Columbia, dried Comfrey leaves contain an NPK ratio of 1.80-0.50-5.30, which is a ratio that is higher than almost all animal manures available on the market today. It also has other nutrients like silica, iron, calcium and magnesium, which are beneficial to many plants.

Comfrey is usually applied as fertilizer in the form of Comfrey compost tea. As a "tea" concentrate, Comfrey's NPK ratio increase even more - to about 8-2.60-20.50. A common way to make compost tea is to stuff and weigh down an old watering can with Comfrey leaves. Wrap the entire can with a black plastic bag to keep rain and insects out. The recommended amount of leaves to use is 5 gallons so keep adding more leaves to the can to top it up. As the liquid concentrate develops in about 3-4 weeks, carefully pour it off into another container.

Another way to harvest your concentrate would be to use two buckets, one placed firmly above the other, with holes drilled into the top bucket. Weigh down your dry, stacked leaves in the top bucket, cover it and allow the liquid concentrate to collect in the lower bucket.

Another method to make Comfrey tea is to stack and weigh down leaves in a container and cover the leaves with water.

Allow the tea to "cook" or infuse for 3-5 weeks. Cooler temperatures will require a longer "cooking" time. *Caution: in all production methods, the concentrate will likely smell very bad. This is normal.*

If you have a smaller garden and need to store the concentrate over winter, store it covered in a dark place. To use the concentrate on your plants, dilute it at 1 part concentrate to 10-20 parts water before application. Comfrey tea is high in readily available potash, which is a good fertilizing option as opposed to inorganic sources, for use on tomatoes, potatoes, peppers and cucumbers.

Note that nitrogen encourages leafy growth while potassium stunts growth while encouraging flower and fruit development. Since the intention of growing most food crops is to bear a lot of fruit, apply your Comfrey fertilizer only after the first flowers have set on your plants.

Foliar Spray

Powdery mildew can be a problem on cucumbers, bee balm and pumpkins. In addition to using the diluted Comfrey tea as a liquid fertilizer, you can also use it as a foliar plant spray. According to a study at the Moscow State University in Russia, *"powdery mildew spores that landed on wheat seedlings sprayed with comfrey tea did not germinate, and the wheat seedlings did not become infected."* The researchers concluded that Comfrey tea helps to activate the wheat seedling's natural defense mechanisms, which makes them more resistant to disease.

The spray should be strained through a fine filter to prevent your sprayer or watering can from clogging up. Make your Comfrey foliar spray even more effective by adding a few drops of a gentle homemade liquid soap. If homemade soap is not available, a brand like Dr. Bronner's will also do the job. The soap helps the spray to stick on the leaves better. Be sure to spray both the top and underside of the leaves.

Mulch

Mulching is another way to use Comfrey as a slow-release fertilizer as it helps to protect the soil surface surrounding the plant. Apply a layer of leaves as mulch around bushes or trees. An easy way to mulch your plants with Comfrey is to plant Comfrey near or by your plants. When you're ready to leaf mulch them, cut the Comfrey leaves down and spread them around the plants that need to be mulched. Be sure, however, to plant Comfrey away from the root zone of young trees because its long tap root may steal nutrients from the growing trees.

Unlike other commonly used carbon-rich mulches like wood chips, Comfrey is high in nitrogen and will therefore not steal it from the soil while breaking down. Use it to mulch fruit trees, berries, flower and fruiting vegetables. Avoid using it to mulch leaf vegetables or root crops as the Comfrey might encourage the plants to bolt (go to seed) early.

Avoid using flowering stems as mulch, which can take root where you did not intend them to. Using leaves that have been dried in the sun for about 2 hours before using them can help to eliminate the problem of the Comfrey taking root. If planting in containers, lay the leaves on the bottom of planting holes in your container. Add a layer of soil on top of the leaves to keep it from burning your plant's roots during the Comfrey's decomposition.

Compost Activator

You can also take advantage of Comfrey's benefits in a compost pile. When added in moderation, Comfrey makes a wonderful addition to a compost pile. Because it breaks down fairly quickly, it will help to speed up the composting process, especially if you have a lot of carbon-rich "brown" compost ingredients such as shredded non-glossy paper or straw.

To make a more effective compost pile, add fresh Comfrey leaves to your "green" nitrogen-rich layers. Green layers normally include fruit and vegetable kitchen scraps. Alternate 6-9 inch green layers between brown ones. Keep the pile moist but not wet. Avoid using too much Comfrey in your pile because the Comfrey may reduce to its liquid-goo concentrate and heat or add too much moisture your compost pile too quickly.

Potting Mixtures

You can also use Comfrey make a Comfrey leaf mold. Compost, on its own, is too dense for planting. Adding leaf mold helps to add air pockets within the compost while making it richer as a planting medium. It also helps to increase water retention in the soil by as much as over 50%.

Making leaf mold is easy but takes time. Make a leaf pile, including the Comfrey leaves, that is at least 3 feet tall and wide, moistening it if it gets dry. You can also fill large plastic bags with moistened leaves to make your leaf mold. Make small holes in the bag to provide airflow and moisten the pile if it gets dry.

The leaf mold should be ready in 6-12 months but you can speed the process up by first shredding the leaves up by running a lawn mower over them. Turning your pile with a garden fork, or shaking your leaf mold bag every few weeks will also help to reduce the decomposition time.

Add your Comfrey leaf mold into your soil or potting mix to help to amend it. You can also apply it to your plants as a mulch.

Food and Fodder

Historically, Comfrey has been used for both food and fodder. While Comfrey appears as a pot herb in some Old World recipes, it is more commonly been used as a tisane in modern times. In the UK, Comfrey has been used for over 200 years as fodder.

In his book, "Russian Comfrey: A Hundred Tons an Acre of Stock Feed or Compost for Farm, Garden or Smallholding",

Lawrence D. Hill, the late British horticulturalist and founder of what is now known as Garden Organic, which now houses the largest body of organic gardeners in the world, praises Comfrey's prolific growth and high protein content.

In his book, Hill reveals that Comfrey produces 3.5 tons of protein compared to the 0.5 tons of protein that soybeans produce in an equivalent crop. Comfrey is also an unusual land plant because it stores Vitamin B-12 from the soil. If you're interested in reading Hill's entire book, you can download the book for free for personal use from the Soil and Health library (http://hyperurl.co/comfreybook).

Comfrey makes for an excellent high-protein fodder which one can use to help save on the cost of using commercially available high-protein feeds. While some livestock may eat Comfrey with relish, others may avoid it because of its prickly leaves. Wilting the leaves before using it as fodder can help to alleviate this problem.

There have been many reports of poultry loving Comfrey but I've found my chickens' reaction to it to be subdued. My geese and donkey, on the other hand, would consume it with gusto. As such, it would be a good idea to keep your Comfrey plants out of reach of your livestock until the plants are established. Consult a livestock vet before using it as fodder.

While Mr. Hill believes that Comfrey "does not make for an attractive source of direct human food," it is nevertheless a potential high protein, easy to grow food source in a survival situation. Bear in mind though, that recent studies have shown that Comfrey can cause liver damage in mice.

Master Herbalist, David Christopher believes that the plant produces toxic alkaloids for the purposes of protecting itself from rodents, and that the benefits of the plant outweighs its toxic components. He notes that mature leaves should be used as a pot herb while young leaves are what are normally used medicinally. While we err on the side of caution and have never consumed Comfrey internally, it may be a food to consider in a starvation situation.

Cultivation

A perennial (that is, the plants will regrow from its roots over the winter,) extremely hardy plant, Comfrey grows best in USDA zones 3-9. However, it is known to withstand the -40°F Russian temperatures through to African heat, which can reach up to 120°F.

While Comfrey grows best in rich, moist loamy soil with a slightly alkaline pH of 6.0-7.0 in full sun, partial shade or heavy shade, it will grow in just about any soil. However, because most strains are deep-rooted, it does not do as well in shallow soil.

Be sure to choose your planting site carefully because where you plant it is where it will stay. Its hardy, deep tap roots that can grow several feet underground, making it hard to eradicate once it's been planted. A new plant can sprout from even a small section of root left in the soil.

Comfrey's hairy leaves can be irritating to the skin so avoid planting it in a location where you may often brush against it. It can grow well on its own but still needs to search for nutrients like nitrogen from the soil. If you are able to plant it near a compost pile, or on an old compost site, it will be able to draw the nutrients that have leached into the soil. Otherwise, it will benefit from regular watering and a dressing of compost or other organic matter at least once a year.

While it may be planted in 5 gallon containers, Comfrey does not generally like to be contained. When planting it in the ground, you can help to control its spreading nature by not cultivating the soil around the Comfrey plant.

Comfrey is an extremely prolific plant. Unless you plant a sterile Bocking variety, Comfrey will propagate by both root and seed. You can prevent non-sterile plants from going to seed by cutting the flower stalks off as they develop. However, I recommend buying sterile varieties to help to keep the plant under control. Each Blocking variety has its own traits and Lawrence Hill's book details the differences between each plant. You can still propagate it by its roots.

Harvesting

Comfrey starts growing in early spring. Once the plant is about 2 feet tall, you can harvest and dry the leaves at any time. However, the best time to harvest is at the end of a sunny but non-humid day when its food value is at its peak.

Cut the plant back to about 2 inches above the crown. If you harvest too early, the plant will not flower. Water your Comfrey plant well after each harvest and replace its mulch if you used any. Fertilizing at this time is optional. Since the leaves are irritating on the skin to most people, it would be a good idea to wear gloves and long sleeves during harvesting.

Harvest on a clear day. Because Comfrey high in protein and moisture, it is important to spread the cuttings out well on a drying spot. If the ground is wet from dew or rain, you might need to dry your cuttings on racks or screens that are raised off the ground. If left in a pile the cuttings may heat up and spoil instead of dry. Allow about 2 days for the cuttings to dry before piling and storing your Comfrey.

Depending on the length of your growing season, you should be able to harvest leaves between 3 to 8 times a year. Each plant produces 3-8 pounds of cuttings per harvest. For best growth, cut the plant monthly to encourage new growth. Healthy Comfrey plants will produce leaves for at least 25 years.

Propagation

Comfrey can grow from non-sterile seeds, root or crown cuttings. Comfrey seeds need to be stratified or winter-chilled before they will germinate. However, it is more difficult to start from seed than from root cuttings because it may take as long as two years before the seeds germinate.

You can also propagate Comfrey from root or crown cuttings. If you plan on just planting a few plants, buy crown cuttings from a local nursery. These cuttings normally have a few eyes and will grow more quickly than root cuttings. Plant crown cuttings 3-6" deep in the ground. However, I think the best option in terms of time and monetary cost is to plant root cuttings as they tend to be less expensive than crown cuttings but will grow and establish much more quickly than from seed.

For optimal planting, prepare your Comfrey bed by removing weeds as thoroughly as possible and dressing the bed with compost or composted manure if possible. Plant the root cuttings about 2-3 feet apart, making sure that the plant shoots are pointed up. Bury the roots about 2-8 inches deep. If you are planting it in clay soil, plant it more shallowly as compared to planting it more deeply in sandy soil. Keep it well watered until the plants are established.

When you have an established plant, you can propagate more by using a spade to splice the plant into two or more pieces. Make sure that roots are part of each divided piece. Replant the pieces as you would a new plant.

Do not harvest in the first year to allow the plants to establish themselves. Remove any flowering stems as well so that the plant can focus its energy on establishing itself. Once established after its first year, the Comfrey plant needs very little care. You might choose to add a light nitrogen application to increase its top growth but I've found it to be unnecessary.

Comfrey may not be the easiest plant to find at many nurseries. At the time of writing, I've found eBay to the the best place to find larger quantities of root cuttings at fairly reasonable prices.

Precautions

There is controversy over the use of Comfrey because it also contains at least 8 pyrrolizidine alkaloids which can cause permanent liver damage or even cause death when ingested. Comfrey cannot be sold for internal use in a number of countries including the US, Canada, Australia, the UK and Germany. Even though I have covered various possible uses for Comfrey in a grid-down situation, **using Comfrey as tea, vegetable or livestock fodder are not recommended by the FDA or the FTC.**

There is varying opinion about the alkaloids being absorbed through the skin from topical use. The general recommendation is that you should not use Comfrey externally for more than 10 days in succession and not more than 4-6 weeks per year. Consult a herbalist or naturopath who can help discuss how herbs can best be applied on an individual basis.

You can find additional information on Comfrey's toxicology from university studies at Cornell University's Department of Animal Science (http://hyperurl.co/cornellcomfrey) and from the University of Maryland Medical Center (http://hyperurl.co/ummcomfrey).

4 ELDERBERRY

Elder or Elderberry (*Sambucus*) is a perennial herbaceous plant which is part of the Adoxaceae family of plants. Also known as flor sauco, tree of music, Danewort, Walewort, it is native to many temperate and subtropical parts of the Northern Hemisphere as well as parts of Asia.

Elder can grow between 5-12 feet tall, with clusters of fragrant, star-shaped flowers blooming in June and July. Its purple-black berries mature in September-October which can be made into preserves, syrup and wine. It prefers to grow in abandoned fields, along roadsides or on the edge of forests.

Uses

Healing Agent

In traditional medicines, all parts of the Elderberry plant are considered important healing agents. Historically, Elder was most commonly used to treat colds, flus and fevers. Dr. Christopher explains that the Elder plant contains potassium chloride, potassium sulphate and potassium phosphate, all of which are present in the Elder flowers. Additionally, potassium nitrate can be found in the leaves. These potassium compounds can help to explain why Elder, especially its flowers, are effective in curing colds and flus.

According to the University of Maryland Medical Center, "the chemicals in elder flower and berries may help reduce swelling in mucous membranes, such as the sinuses, and help relieve nasal congestion. Elder may have anti-inflammatory, antiviral, and anti-cancer properties."

Elderberry Syrup

Ingredients

1. 1/2 cup dried Elderberries
2. 3 cups filtered water
3. 1/2 to 1 cup raw unfiltered honey (if you don't have bees, you can get it from most Costcos or natural foods stores)
4. 1 cinnamon stick (optional)
5. 1 clove or 1/4 tsp clove powder (optional)
6. 1 thin slice of ginger or 1/2 tsp ginger powder (optional)

Method

1. In a clean saucepan, bring the Elderberries and spices in the water to a boil.
2. Lower the heat and simmer for about 30 minutes.
3. Remove from heat.
4. Strain the solids out.
5. When the liquid is slightly cool, add the honey and mix well.
6. Allow the mixture to cool before pouring it into a glass bottle.
7. Store in the refrigerator.

The mixture should keep for about 2 months in the fridge. Dr. Christopher suggested a dosage of 1/2 tsp to 1 tsp daily for children and 1/2 Tbsp to 1 Tbsp for adults to help to boost the immune system. For those who already have a cold, he upped the daily dose to every 2-3 hours until the symptoms disappeared.

Elder Leaf Ointment

Elder leaves are used for making salves and oils which can be used to make ointments to help to treat sprains, bruises, sunburns, rashes and wounds.

Ingredients

1. 4 oz crushed Elderberry leaves
2. 6 oz liquid organic coconut oil (use melted lard or other animal fat in times of crisis)
3. 2 tsp Eucalyptol or Eucalyptus oil (omit if it is unavailable)

Method

1. Place the Elder leaves and oil in a roasting pan.
2. Place the pan in an oven at medium heat.
3. Stir the leaves in the oil until they lose their color and turn crisp.
4. Remove from the heat and strain the oil through a cheesecloth.
5. Add the Eucalyptol to the oil and stir well.
6. Pour into a glass jar and allow to cool before storing.

Oil of Elder Leaves

Oil of Elder leaves is slightly easier to make and is normally used on burns and wounds.

Method

Simmer one part Elder leaves in 3 parts of olive oil until the leaves turn crisp. Allow the oil to cool a little, strain and bottle it. Allow it to cool completely before storing.

Elderberry Tisane

Simmer elderberry flowers for 10 minutes. The resulting tisane is said to ease eye twitching and inflammation when a piece of cotton saturated in Elderberry tisane is applied on closed eyelids. The tisane can also be used as a wash for dry skin. It can also be enjoyed as a fragrant beverage.

-   *Recipes adapted from the Master Herbalist Guide by Dr. Christopher*

Pest Deterrent

While I have no personal anecdotes on the effectiveness of Elder as a pest deterrent, Elder has historically been used to deter pests. Dried Elder leaves, mixed with grain before storage is said to deter mice, moles and weevils. In Old Europe, Elder was planted on each corner of the house to deter mice from entering.

Food

Elder flowers and berries can be collected and preserved by drying from July to October, depending on which part of the country you're in. Elderberries are most commonly used to make jams, jellies, pie fillings, sauces and wine. However, the flowers can also be used to make light pancakes and fritters.

Elderflower Fritters

Ingredients

1. Elderflower clusters
2. 1 c all-purpose flour, sifted
3. 1 Tbsp sugar
4. 1 tsp baking powder
5. 2 eggs
6. 1/2 c milk

Method

1. Wash and drain the flower clusters.
2. Beat all the ingredients except the flower clusters together until you produce a batter.
3. Heat the oil to 375°F.
4. Dip the flower clusters into the batter.
5. Fry the battered flower clusters in the oil for 4 minutes or until they are golden brown.
6. Drain on a paper towel.
7. Roll in granulated sugar (optional).
8. Serve hot.

- *Recipe adapted from Food.com*

Elderberry Wine

Ingredients

1. 1 quart firmly packed blossoms, separated from the stems
2. 3 gallons water
3. 9 lb sugar
4. 3 lb seedless raisins, chopped
5. 1/2 c strained lemon juice (about 4 lemons)
6. 1 cake compressed yeast

Method

1. Boil the sugar in water for about 5 minutes until it becomes a thin syrup.
2. Mix the blossoms in well.
3. Allow the liquid to cool to lukewarm temperature.
4. Add the rest of the ingredients.
5. Allow the mixture to stand for 6 days in a non-reactive container, stirring it 3 times a day.
6. Strain the wine, date the container and allow it to age for at least 6 months, preferably 12.
7. Pour the final liquid into glass bottles and cap. Label and date the bottles.

- *Recipe adapted from Faith B. Lasher on Mother Earth News*

Elderberry Jelly

Ingredients

1. 3 pounds Elderberries
2. Juice of 1 lemon
3. 1 box fruit pectin
4. 4 1/2 cups sugar
5. Water

Method

1. In a saucepan, heat the berries on low heat until the juice starts to flow.
2. Simmer for 15 minutes
3. Strain the liquid through double layers of cheesecloth into another saucepan.
4. Mix in the lemon juice.
5. Add enough water to make up 3 cups of liquid.
6. Add the pectin.
7. Bring the mixture to a boil and stir in the sugar.
8. Allow to cool before using.

- *Recipe by Faith B. Lasher on Mother Earth News*

Note: This recipe has not been tested for safe canning. For safe canning recipes, refer to the most recent Ball Canning or University Extension Office publications.

Pontack - Elderberry Sauce

An old English recipe, this Elderberry sauce goes well with wild game.

Ingredients

1. 2 pounds fresh Elderberries, or 12 ounces dried Elderberries
2. 4 cups cider vinegar
3. 1 pound shallots, minced
4. 10 cloves
5. 10 allspice berries
6. 1 teaspoon nutmeg
7. 2 tablespoons cracked black peppercorns
8. 1 teaspoon salt

Method

1. Clean the Elderberries and remove all stems and debris.
2. Place the Elderberries and vinegar in an oven-proof dish.
3. Cook the mixture for 4-6 hours at 250°F.
4. Carefully remove the pan from the oven and strain the liquid into a clean saucepan.
5. Allow the berries to cool and use your hands to squeeze as much juice from the berries as possible into a pot.
6. Discard/compost the spent berries.
7. Add the remaining ingredients and simmer on low heat for about 25 minutes.

8. Strain out the spices.
9. Bring the sauce to a boil for 5 minutes.

- *Recipe adapted from The River Cottage Preserves by Pam Corbin*

Note: This recipe has not been tested for safe canning. For safe canning recipes, refer to the most recent Ball Canning or University Extension Office publications.

Wildlife Attractant

Fancy some meat to go with that Elderberry sauce? According to the USDA, Elderberry plants attract a host of wildlife. If planted along streams, their roots help to stabilize banks and help to provide a habitat for fish and other aquatic creatures. Elder foliage and berries attract many wild game and birds including pheasants, grouse, pigeons, bears, deer, elk and moose.

Developing a Elderberry habitat will help to lure wild birds and game, which will provide an additional meat source in a bug-in situation. Of course, you will also need to know how to trap or hunt and properly butcher your game.

Cultivation

According to Gardening.org, Elderberry fruits are best when you plant at least 2 varieties of plants within 60 feet of each other. American varieties like Adams, Johns, York and Nova tend to be better fruit producers as compared to European Elderberry varieties, which are more ornamental.

Elderberries are hardy perennials that will grow in Zones 3-10. They prefer to grow in full or partial sun. Elderberries will grow in various soil types and pH levels. However, they grow best in slightly acidic, nutrient-rich, consistently moist but well draining soil.

Amend clay soils with compost before planting. You may need to plant Elderberries in raised beds to ensure proper drainage if you are planting on heavy clay soils. Depending on the variety, space plants 6-10 feet apart. Fertilize the plants annually with compost for best growing results. Because Elderberries have shallow roots, it is a good idea to mulch around the plants using straw or wood chips. Mulching will also help to keep weeds under control and prevent water loss from surface evaporation.

Elderberries send suckers out freely. These suckers become new branches every season which will fruit heavily in their second or third year. After 3 years, the branches become less productive. At this time, prune them in late winter but leave about equal numbers of first, second and third year branches. Remove any dead, diseased or broken branches. Pruning will also help to control cane borers, which can infect older branches.

Harvesting

Harvest Elderberry flowers around July and Elder fruit from August to October, depending on the growing region and variety. Pick the flowers when they are shedding pollen, on a sunny day. Wait for the Elderberries to be ripe and dark purple before harvesting.

Collect the berries by cutting off the entire cluster and stripping the berries into a bowl. Refrigerate them after harvesting and process the berries as soon as possible because they do not store well, especially at room temperature.

Propagation

Seeds

According to the USDA, Elderberries grow best from seed. Elderberry produces a good seed crop almost every year. Collect the elderberry fruits when ripe and spread them in thin layers to dry.

There are a couple of ways to harvest the seeds. The easiest method is to crush and dry the berries without separating the seeds from the pulp. You can also run the berries through a macerator with water (or a fruit blender if you're working with a smaller amount of berries). The pulp and seeds that are not viable will float, allowing you to harvest the viable seeds that settle. Allow it to air dry. Elderberry seeds will remain viable for several years if stored dry at 41°F and may last for up to 16 years.

Elder seeds have a hard seed coat and therefore need to be sown in fall or stratified for 3-5 months before sowing in spring. Without pretreatment, germination may be delayed by 2 to 5 years. They can be sown in the fall following the collection or stratified and sown in spring.

To stratify seeds, you can use sifted peat moss which works well for small seeds. Dampen the moss and add one part horticultural sand or vermiculite to four parts peat moss to improve soil aeration.

In a small bowl, place a handful of this soilless mix and make a large depression in the center. Add as many seeds as you wish in the depression. Cover it with more mix then remove the seeds in the mixture from the boil, gently squeezing out the excess moisture. Be careful not to compact it.

Place your seed/soil-less mix into a ziplock bag and label it with the plant name and date. Leave it in a warm place like on a seed heating mat or on top of the refrigerator for 3 days. Place the bag in the coldest area of the fridge (but not the freezer), which is usually in the meat drawer. Shake the bag once or twice a week to keep it aerated. After keeping the seeds chilled for 3-5 months, sow the seeds in the soil-less mix directly into 3 inch deep pots filled with seed-starting mix.

Elder seeds may also be warm stratified for 2 months in the greenhouse using a mixture of peat, vermiculite and sand at 70 - 85°F. Place the seeds close to the soil surface in flats in the greenhouse before potting them in 3 inch deep pots. Allow the seeds to grow in a warm, sunny location until it is ready to be transplanted outdoors, when they are 6-8 months old.

You can also plant the seeds in fall and allow them to stratify naturally over the winter. Bear in mind that in either case, the germination will usually not be complete until the second spring. Sow the seeds about 1/4 inch deep and cover with about 3/8 inch of sawdust mulch. In drier planting sites, keep the seeds or seedlings well watered until they are established. If the Elderberry plants are planted on a moist site, irrigation may not be needed in the fall.

Cuttings

You can also use hardwood cuttings from previous season's growth to propagate elderberry plants. Even though cuttings tend to have a lower survival rate than plants established from seeds, they tend to grow faster when successfully established.

To make cuttings, take cuttings at least 10 inches long with at least two side shoots from older wood, preferably without flowers. Take heel cuttings from older wood, that is, cut off the shoot with a sliver of the main stem attached such that it forms a heel shape.

Place the cuttings in 4" pots filled with perlite and peat, keeping the plants moist. You will experience a high mortality rate during this transplant process so be very gentle with its delicate roots.

Precautions

Consuming Elderberries raw or undried can result in vomiting and diarrhea. Unripe berries are toxic and may cause nausea. Only blue and purple Elderberries are edible. **Do not consume red berries of other species as they are toxic and should not be gathered.**

Elderberry fruits may be toxic to chickens. Elderberry leaves and stems contain cyanide and can cause poisoning if ingested. Cattle may also refuse to eat elder leaves. Consult a livestock veterinarian before using Elder on your livestock.

5 GARLIC

With thousands of years of history of human use, Garlic (*Allium sativum; Liliaceae*) needs little introduction. However, because Garlic has remarkable curative properties, can be used as a food, and can be grown in most climates, it is important that I include this wonderful plant in this book. Although it is usually grown as an annual, it is a perennial bulbous plant.

Native to central Asia, Garlic has long, narrow grass-like leaves. Whitish flowers are located at the end of their stalks, which grow out from bulbs at the base. The bulbs consists of 4-20 bulblets or cloves that are grouped together, each encased in a thin, white papery membrane. The Garlic bulb has been used since historical times for both food and medicine while its green scapes can be used for food.

Uses

Healing Agent

Garlic has natural antiseptic and antibacterial properties. In both World War I and II, soldiers were given Garlic to prevent gangrene. To help to prevent wound infection, fresh raw Garlic juice was diluted with water and applied onto wounds using sterilized sphagnum moss.

According to the University of Maryland Medical Center, Garlic is rich in antioxidants which can help to fight off free radicals that build up in the body. Free radicals may contribute to heart disease, cancer, and Alzheimer's disease.

Eating Garlic regularly may help to protect against these diseases as well as help to prevent heart disease, high cholesterol, high blood pressure, and to boost the immune system. Consuming Garlic may also help to prevent colds and to make the symptoms go away more quickly.

According to German researchers, Garlic is most effective when consumed crushed (not sliced) in a fresh, raw form. The antibacterial action becomes weaker after being refrigerated for over a week and after boiling for 10 minutes. The study also noted that the beneficial organic sulphur contents turns into a harmful inorganic sulphur when garlic is cooked at above 130°F.

Four Thieves Vinegar

According to French folklore, sometime between the 14th and 18th centuries, four grave robbers in Marseilles spent their nights robbing the bodies of victims of The Black Death during a plague. They were said to have been able to escape the ravages of the plague because they'd doused face masks, and themselves, in a strong antibacterial and antiviral herbal vinegar.

Upon their capture, they were able to lessen their sentence from burning at the stake to a hanging by revealing the secret to their immunity. Their secret was what is now normally known as the Four Thieves Vinegar. While there are many variations as to how to make Four Thieves Vinegar, modern day recipes usually include vinegar, garlic, lavender, sage, thyme, mint, wormwood, rue and/or rosemary.

While its use to prevent the plague is not a statement approved by the FDA, nor have I personally had any experience in its use as a plague preventative, today's Four Thieves Vinegar is normally applied by spray bottle and used as a natural sterilizing agent to clean kitchen and bathroom surfaces. I suggest using distilled white vinegar if you plan to use the Four Thieves for cleaning.

You can also use apple cider vinegar but the resulting vinegar will not last as long. However, apple cider vinegar would be a preferred choice if you plan on consuming it. When the apple cider vinegar version of Four Thieves Vinegar is mixed with extra virgin olive oil and salt and pepper to taste it makes a tasty vinaigrette.

Ingredients

1. 4 cloves of Garlic, raw (peeled and crushed)
2. 1 Tbsp Sage leaves
3. 1 tsp Lavender flowers
4. 1 tsp Rosemary leaves
5. 1/2 tsp Thyme leaves
6. 16 oz vinegar

Method

1. Place the herbs in a pint jar.
2. Fill the jar to the top with gently warmed (but not boiled) vinegar.
3. Cover the jar top with a plastic lid or use a piece of natural parchment paper to separate the jar from a metal lid.

4. Allow the extract to sit undisturbed for 4 weeks.
5. Strain the extract into a clean glass jar and cover.

- *Recipe adapted from Mountain Rose Herbs*

Garlic Syrup

For asthma, coughs and tuberculosis, Dr. Christopher developed a Garlic syrup remedy.

Ingredients

1. 1 lb fresh Garlic, peeled and minced
2. 1 pint food grade vegetable glycerine
3. 3 lbs honey, preferably organic and raw
4. 1:1 parts of vinegar and distilled water

Method

1. Add the Garlic into a clean, wide mouthed glass jar.
2. Add enough of the 1:1 part vinegar to distilled water to cover the Garlic.
3. Cover tightly, shake well and allow the jar to stand in a cool place for 4 days, shaking once or twice a day.
4. Add the vegetable glycerine to the infusion, shake well.
5. Allow the mixture to stand for a day.
6. Strain the liquid into another large enough clean jar through a linen or muslin cloth, making sure to apply enough pressure to draw as much liquid out as possible.
7. Add the honey to the strained liquid and stir until fully blended.

8. Store in tightly sealed clean glass jars in a cool dry place.

Dosage

For asthma and coughs, Dr. Christopher recommended a dosage of 1 tsp of Garlic syrup, with or without water every 15 minutes until the spasms subside then 1 tsp of the syrup every 2-3 hours for the rest of the day. After that, he suggested taking 1 tsp of the syrup 3-4 times a day.

For tuberculosis, dyspnea and cardiac asthma Dr. Christopher's suggested dosage was 1 tsp to 1 Tbsp of Garlic syrup taken 3-4 times a day between meals.

He halved the dosage for children 8-15 years old, quartered the dosage and diluted it with a little water or honey for children aged 5-8 and used 1/8th the dose for children between 1 to 4 years old.

Dr. Christopher's Anti-Plague Super Garlic Immune Formula

Since plagues and epidemics can occur at any time, it would be to the serious prepper's benefit to make this formula in advance and store it, being thankful if you never have to use it. Dr. Christopher said that it has been used with good results for many ailments.

Ingredients

1. 8 parts apple cider vinegar
2. 5 parts food grade vegetable glycerine
3. 5 parts honey
4. 2 parts fresh Garlic juice
5. 2 parts Comfrey root concentrate
6. 1 part Wormwood concentrate
7. 1 part Lobelia leaf or seed concentrate
8. 1 part Oak bark concentrate
9. 1 part Black Walnut bark concentrate
10. 1 part Mullein leaf concentrate
11. 1 part Skullcap leaf concentrate
12. 1 part Uva Ursi, hydrangea or gravel root concentrate
13. 1 part Marshmallow root concentrate

Make each concentrate separately. To make concentrates, soak the respective herb for at least 4 hours in enough distilled water to cover it completely. After soaking, add more distilled water to make 16 oz or 0.5 liters of water per 4 oz or 113g herb.

Using either a glass, porcelain or stainless steel pot, simmer the herb on very low heat in a covered pan. Do not use aluminum, teflon or cracked porcelain for this process. You can also use an uncovered double boiler for this process. Allow the liquid to simmer down to a quarter of its original volume (you should get 4 oz of final concentrate).

Mix the liquid ingredients well only after all the concentrates are prepared.

Dosage

Dr. Christopher used a dosage of 1 tsp 3 times a day as a preventative or 1 Tbsp every half an hour if infected.

Pesticide / Pest Deterrent

You can use Garlic to make a simple organic pest deterrent by infusing crushed Garlic in water. To make a dilute pesticide, pour 1 gallon of boiling water over 6 cloves of crushed Garlic. Allow it to steep overnight before using it.

You can increase the concentration by using up to 2 full bulbs of Garlic blended in 1/2 cup of water. To make the infusion more potent, you can also add crushed Cayenne pepper to the mix before pouring the boiling water on the garlic. **Use gloves and goggles when making this.** Allow the infusion to steep overnight, squeeze and strain the liquid into a spray bottle.

Apply the Garlic spray once every few days or weekly as a pest deterrent. Remember to spray the leaf bottoms, which harbor many pests. Reapply the spray after plant watering or after a rain.

Fish Bait

Whether you're in a homesteading or survival situation, knowing that you can use Garlic to bait most bottom feeding fish like catfish and carp is helpful if you need to add more food to your plate.

To make bottom-feeder Garlic bait, add garlic powder or minced fresh Garlic to blended food scraps. The consistency of the final product should be like that of dough. Add water to the mixture if it's too dry to hold together. Shape the mixture into bait-sized balls and freeze them. Allow your Garlic-scrap bait to thaw before use.

Food

Garlic needs little introduction when it comes to using it in food. It is added to many Asian, Middle Eastern, North African, Southern European and parts of South and Central American cuisine. Both the bulbs and the scapes (the green stems) can be used as food. Both are usually chopped up and added into dishes for additional flavor. However, Garlic sometimes features as the main ingredient in a dish.

Pickled Garlic

Pickled garlic is a great way to serve Garlic as a dish, side dish or as a condiment.

Ingredients

1. 3 lbs peeled whole Garlic cloves
2. 6 cups white wine vinegar (or any vinegar of your choice)
3. 1 Tbsp pickling salt
4. 1/2 cup sugar
5. 1 tsp dried Oregano (optional)
6. 2 tsp dried red pepper flakes (optional)

Method

1. On a stove top, bring a large pot of water to a rolling boil.
2. Fill another large bowl with ice and fill halfway with water.
3. Place all the Garlic in the boiling water and blanch for 1 minute. (Do not wait for the water to boil before starting your time.)
4. Drain the Garlic and immerse it immediately in the ice water bath.
5. Allow the Garlic to cool entirely.
6. Bring the rest of the ingredients to a boil in a large non-reactive pot until the salt and sugar is all dissolved.
7. Fill a clean glass jar with the Garlic and cover them with the vinegar solution.

8. Cover the jar with a non-reactive lid.
9. Allow the Garlic to pickle for 3-4 weeks in the refrigerator before consumption.
10. You may also add other dried herbs or spices to this pickle recipe according to taste.

- *Recipe adapted from Food.com*

Honeyed Garlic *(Ninniku Hachimitsu-zuke)*

This is a very easy preservation method that allows you to preserve your Garlic cloves in a delicious manner. Honeyed Garlic is also used as a herbal remedy against colds and flus because of its antibacterial and antiviral properties. It also makes a delicious addition to Asian stir fries.

If you use a tube garlic peeler, you should be able to reduce the time and labor needed to peel garlic. Tube garlic peelers cost about $2-$8 on Amazon or other retailers and are worth the investment if you have a lot of garlic to process.

You can also peel Garlic cloves by placing them in a jar. Twirl the cloves around in the covered jar until the peels fall off.

Ingredients

1. Garlic cloves, peeled
2. Enough raw honey, preferable organic, to cover the Garlic cloves

Method

1. Only use fresh Garlic cloves. Do not use garlic cloves that are dry/dried up, bruised, rotting or already sprouting.
2. Fill a clean glass jar with Garlic cloves, leaving about 1-2 inches of headspaoo.
3. Cover the Garlic cloves with the honey, leaving at least 1 inch of headspace from the top of the jar.
4. The Garlic will float to the top.

5. Keep the Garlic cloves covered in honey by weighing it down with a clean, non-reactive weight, or by inverting the jar every day (this can get messy). You can also use a clean spoon to push the Garlic into the honey every day to keep it coated in honey.
6. Cover the jar loosely to allow the air to vent out during fermentation.
7. Optional but recommended: place a small bowl or dish under the jar to prevent the honey from making a mess if it overflows during the ferment.
8. Allow the Garlic to ferment for at least a month.
9. The Garlic is ready when they sink in the honey. However, they will continue to cure and sweeten over time.

- *Recipe by Quick & Easy Tsukemono: Japanese Pickling Recipes*

Cultivation

There are two general kinds of Garlic: hardneck and softneck. Hardnecks tend to fare better in cold climates and have a small number of cloves arranged around the main stem. The cloves are easier to peel and have a stronger flavor. Most grocery store Garlic varieties are hardneck.

Softnecks on the other hand, produce smaller cloves and grow in artichoke-like layers. They are milder in flavor but harder to peel. They tend to store better and fare better in milder climates. However, the issue of hardneck versus softneck hardiness is very general because Garlics are very adaptable.

Garlics grow best in Zones 3-8 in neutral to slightly acidic soil in full sun. The soil should be nutrient-rich, loamy and well-draining. While you can plant Garlic in spring, as soon as the ground is worked, the cloves tend to not bulb out. Instead, the cloves often merely grow bigger if planted in spring. If the cloves bulb out, the bulbs tend to be smaller. The best time to plant Garlic is in fall.

Amend your planting area by first broadcasting clover or alfalfa seeds then covering them with a thin layer of soil on your planned garlic patch in mid-summer. Till the green manure under when it reaches about 2 inches in height.

You can also add grass clippings to your planned garlic bed about a month before you plant the Garlic. Water the planting bed several weeks before planting to encourage any weed seeds to sprout. Once the weeds have sprouted, carefully till them under to kill them. Spread alfalfa pellets on the patch just before you plant the Garlic. Alfalfa pellets are often sold as horse feed at ranch and livestock feed supply stores.

Garlics are grown from cloves. However, garlic heads purchased from the grocery store will likely not be suited for planting in your area. You can, however, plant cloves from garlic heads purchased at local farmer's markets, assuming that the garlics are locally grown. You can also buy garlic for planting from local nurseries or from online sources although the latter tends to be the most expensive option.

Plant the cloves about a month before the ground freezes. In areas that experience long hard frosts, plant the cloves about 6-8 weeks before the ground freezes. Carefully break the cloves apart before planting, leaving the clove's papery sheath intact. Plant only the largest cloves because final bulb size depends on the original clove's size. Save the smaller cloves for consumption and discard cloves that are decayed or moldy.

Plant the cloves upright in 3-inch furrows about 2 inches deep and 4-6 inches apart with their pointy end facing upwards. Water well and mulch the garlic bed with 3-6 inches of loose organic mulch like straw or hay. Mulch more thickly if you live in a cold region. Mulching will help to retain water and keep weeds out. Leave the bed alone over winter.

In spring, remove the mulch after the threat of frost has passed. Water the bed if it appears dry and fertilize when the stiff green stems growing from the mature plant, also called garlic scapes, appear. Cut off the scapes. Not only are they good in stir fries or braised in olive oil, cutting the scapes off will also make the garlic bulbs grow bigger. Only hardneck varieties produce scapes. Fertilize as needed. Garlic is a heavy nitrogen feeder and its leaves yellowing is a sign of a nitrogen deficiency.

Keep the bed weeded and consistently moist (every 3-5 days) but not wet, which can rot the garlic. Reduce waterings and allow the soil to dry out in mid-summer when the leaves start to die back. This process will toughen the skin on the garlic bulbs.

Harvesting

It is time to harvest when all but 4-5 leaves are brown. On a cloudy day, carefully lift the bulbs using a fork or shovel. Resist the urge to pull them out because you will run the risk of bruising them. The bulb wrappers should not disintegrate and the bulb should not be small. Weak wrappers or small bulbs are a sign that the garlic was dug up prematurely. Brush the excess soil from the bulbs and place them in a shady staging area where you can remove any additional soil from the Garlic.

Cure the Garlic by tying them into small bundles and hanging them to dry in a well-ventilated place. The curing process takes about 6 weeks. Trim the roots and stems and store the bulbs in a cool, dry place. Do not store them in moist or humid areas. The garlic can be consumed at any time after it is harvested.

Propagation

To propagate Garlic, save the largest, well-formed bulbs to replant in fall.

Precautions

The USDA recognizes Garlic as GRAS (generally recognized as safe). However, side effects of Garlic can include bad breath, body odor, bloating and upset stomach. Handling too much Garlic may cause a stinging sensation and in extreme cases, may cause lesions. Rarer side effects include allergies, headaches, fatigue and dizziness. Some people may be allergic to Garlic.

Garlic acts like a blood thinner and may react with other herbs, supplements or medications. Consuming medical amounts of Garlic may cause problems for people with clotting disorders.

6 MARSHMALLOW

Human use of Marshmallows (*Althaea officinalis; Malvaceae*) goes as far back as the ancient Egyptians and Romans. However, it was not until around the early 19th century, when the French started whipping up the sap extracted from the Marshmallow root and sweetening it, that the predecessor to today's sweet confection was born. Far removed from its sugary namesake, the Marshmallow's genus name hints of its curative prowess. *Althaea* is derived from the Greek word, *altho*, which means to cure.

The Marshmallow plant is a perennial plant which is native to Europe, Northern Africa and Western Asia. Sometimes also referred to as "cheesies" or "Bread and Butter" because their small, round seed pods are reminiscent of cheese wheels. The Marshmallow plant normally hugs the ground in mat-like manner. However, in good growing conditions, they can reach heights of 3-4 feet.

The 2-3 inch ovate-cordate leaves are irregularly toothed on the edges. Although other mallows may also be referred to as Marshmallows, the true Marshmallow is distinguished by the numerous divisions of the outer calyx (six to nine cleft), by the greyish down that covers the stems and foliage thickly. It is also distinguished by the numerous panicles of blush-colored flowers, which are paler than those the common mallow.

The five-petaled flowers bloom between August and September. The roots are tough but pliant; thick, long and tapering. They are tan on the outside but white and fibrous within. The entire plant contains a mild, healing gummy substance called mucilage, with the highest concentrations of mucilage found in its roots.

I rank Marshmallow highly in this list of medicinal plants for the homesteader and/or prepper because it has powerful healing properties, makes for a nutritious and palatable dish and grows abundantly in most climates and altitudes across North America.

Uses

Healing Agent

It is mostly the leaves and roots of Marshmallow that are used for medicinal purposes. Its gummy mucilage which has anti-inflammatory flavonoids that line and coat membranes. It has been used to help relieve coughs and bronchitis. It is also used to relieve diarrhea, stomach ulcers, constipation and stones in the urinary tract.

Marshmallow roots are either brewed in cold water to make a tea, or eaten raw and have been used as a diuretic and a kidney healer. Brewing in cold water preserves the Marshmallow's mucilaginous properties.

Like the Plantain (Plantago, not the banana-like fruit) plant, Marshmallow leaves can be turned into a poultice to be applied directly onto the skin for insect bites and stings. Marshmallow roots can also be mashed and applied directly to the skin for skin ulcers and abscesses. Ointments containing Marshmallow root can also be used to help heal chapped skin.

A Marshmallow infusion is where its roots are steeped in lukewarm water overnight. After the roots are strained out, the resulting infusion has been used as a mouthwash for canker sores and other painful mouth conditions, as a heartburn remedy or as a skin wash for topical treatment for burns and wounds. Marshmallow infusions have also been used to soothe skin rashes and irritations.

Although King's American Dispensatory mentions in 1898 that "marshmallow root is very useful in the form of poultice, to discuss painful, inflammatory tumors, and swellings of every kind, whether the consequence of wounds, bruises, burns, scalds, or poisons; and has, when thus applied, had a happy effect in preventing the occurrence of gangrene. The infusion or decoction may be freely administered", Marshmallow's ability to prevent and possibly even cure gangrene is not widely discussed amongst present-day herbalists.

In his time, Dr. Christopher often used Marshmallow to help to prevent gangrene. He notes many successes using Marshmallow to save his patients from limb amputation. Dr. Christopher's method of curing gangrene consisted of rinsing clean bushels of Marshmallow plants and roots and simmering them in large, non-reactive (stainless steel or unchipped enamel) pots. Do not use copper or aluminum. He then added at least an ounce of Cayenne pepper to the tea.

He then immersed the infected area or limb in the Marshmallow tea for 30 minutes. The tea should be as hot as the skin can bear without scalding it. After 30 minutes, he immersed the infected area in ice cold water for 5 minutes before re-immersing the infected area to a fresh hot Marshmallow and Cayenne tea for 30 minutes.

The process was then repeated all day long until he alleviated the extreme pain enough to apply the same very hot Marshmallow and Cayenne tea hot pad on the infected area. To make the hot pad, soak a tea towel in the Marshmallow and Cayenne tea such that the towel is wet but not dripping. He placed the hot pad on the infected area overnight, keeping it warm with a hot water bottle. Only use a moist (never dry) heat source to keep the pad warm.

Next, he continued the soaking process the next day and had his patient drink three cups of Marshmallow root tea a day until the infection is healed. Dr. Christopher also recommended a raw or low-heated vegan diet following the healing.

Food

Marshmallow contains high quality proteins and is rich in calcium, iron, potassium, magnesium as well as vitamin C. Given that the Marshmallow plant grows easily and abundantly in a wide range of conditions, it makes for an excellent survival food crop.

Marshmallow leaves produce a mucus similar to that of okra which can be used as a soup thickener. The Marshmallow mucilage is concentrated in its roots and when boiled in water, the roots release a thick mucus that can be beaten to make a meringue-like egg substitute.

The flowers and mildly-flavored leaves can be chopped finely (to counter their hairiness), consumed raw and added to salads. The Marshmallow fruits can be used as a caper substitute. Because of its mucilaginous nature, Marshmallow is best mixed with other vegetables rather than consumed on its own, which can be too slimy to be palatable.

According to "A Modern Herbal" by Margaret Grieve, the roots have been used in difficult times to make a palatable dish of first boiled, then fried, roots with onions. When dried, the Marshmallow leaves and flowers can also be used to make tisanes.

Cultivation

Erfurt Marshmallow (*Althea officinalis 'Erfurter'*) is a good variety to consider because it has a higher mucilage content and is available from Richter's Herbs (http://hyperurl.co/marshmallowseeds).

Marshmallow plants are frost-hardy perennials that will grow in Zones 3-9. They prefer to grow in full or partial sun. Marshmallow will grow in sandy, loamy or clay soil types, in both acidic and alkaline soils as well as in saline soil but they grow best in a sunny location with rich moist soil. They will however, tolerate dry conditions.

Marshmallow can be cultivated from seeds or from cuttings. Planting seeds can be as easy as scattering seeds in a location that does not have already have Marshmallow plants growing. However, optimal planting calls for direct sowing seeds about an inch deep in fall. Seeds can be started in spring but need to be stratified for 3-4 weeks before planting. To stratify seeds, mix the seeds in a moist but not wet planting medium and place the mixture in a ziplock bag in the fridge. Shake the bag occasionally during the stratification process.

You can also sow the seeds in flats and then placing the entire flat in a refrigerator. Keep the seeds moist until they germinate. The seeds should be transplanted into larger containers as soon as they start to germinate. Allow the seedlings to grow indoors for a few weeks before transplanting them 18-24 inches apart outside in late spring.

Even though Marshmallow will tolerate dry spells, do not allow them to dry out. It's best to keep the Marshmallow patch well-watered for healthy plants. While not necessary, you may choose to fertilize the plants with a side dressing of worm castings or well composted animal manure every 2-3 years.

Harvesting

Marshmallow plants are slower to mature and will only begin to flower in August or September of their second year. It will take a few years before the roots are large enough to harvest for medicinal purposes. The roots are best harvested by

digging them up with a spade on a dry day in late fall, when the mucilage content is higher.

The roots can be used fresh or dried. To dry the roots, first wash them, then, if they are large roots, cut or slice them. Dry the roots on screens in a well-ventilated shaded area that is around 85-95°F. Do not however, allow the roots to dry at temperatures above 104°F. The roots are dried when they are hard and brittle to the touch. If it feels leathery, it needs to be dried more.

You can harvest the leaves at any time to make a fresh poultice. For longer term storage, flowers and leaves should be collected between late summer to early fall by cutting or plucking. Tie the leaves up in bunches and hang them up to dry in a shaded but well-ventilated area. Again, the leaves are dry when they are brittle to the touch. Store the dried plants in an air-tight container in a cool, dry place.

Propagation

In late summer, wait until the seed pods are dry and ready to burst open. On a clear day, collect the seeds into an envelope and store them a cool, dry, dark location. Marshmallow can also be propagated by root cuttings. Dig up and divide the roots in spring, before the plants sprout, or in fall, after the plant has died back.

Use a shovel or a sharp knife to make your root divisions, allowing the exposed cut areas to dry and cure before re-potting them. Keep the root divisions potted in a well-watered growing medium under a cold frame until the plants are strong enough to be transplanted into their permanent location.

Precautions

According to the University of Maryland Medical Center, Marshmallow is generally regarded as safe. It has no reported side effects but may interact with other herbs, supplements or medications to trigger side effects.

Because Marshmallow coats the stomach lining, it should only be taken several hours before or after taking other herbs or medication. People with diabetes, have allergies, on lithium, who are pregnant or are taking other medications or herbs should consult their healthcare provider before using Marshmallow.

7 PEPPERMINT

An ancient herb prized by the ancient Egyptians, Greeks and Romans and frequently mentioned by Hippocrites, Peppermint (*Mentha piperita; Labiatae*) is a perennial herbaceous plant that needs little introduction. Native to Europe and the Middle East, it is now widespread in many parts of the world.

A hybrid plant, Peppermint seeds are usually sterile. The plant propagates from its wide spreading, fleshy rhizomes, growing to heights as tall as 3 feet. However, it tends to exhibit a creeping growth pattern. The slightly fuzzy, dark-green leaves with reddish veins range between 1.5-3.5 inches long and around 1 inch wide on average. Peppermint flowers from mid to late summer, bearing small (0.2-0.3 inches) purple flowers that grow in whorls around the stem.

Uses

Healing Agent

Peppermint is a pungent mint and is commonly used as a sedative to help to calm nerves and aid in relaxation and sleep. Peppermint is often used as a remedy for colds and the flu. A hot tisane of equal parts of Peppermint and Elder flowers; or an infusion of Peppermint alone is also used to break fevers.

Peppermint tea consumed after a meal may help to prevent flatulence. Dr. Christopher also suggested that consuming peppermint tea regularly instead of coffee or regular tea will help to improve general digestion. It may also help to ease nausea, queasy stomach, stomach pain stemming from pockets of gas and infant colic. For small infants unable to consume Peppermint tea, slightly warmed leaves placed on the infant's stomach is said to also help.

A strong Peppermint tea infusion coupled with rest has also been used in place of aspirin or other inorganic painkillers to help to relieve pain. According to the late naturopath, Dr. Shook, Peppermint can even be used to relieve severe pain.

Dr. Shook's Peppermint Decoction for Severe Pain

Dr. Shook administered his Peppermint decoction to people suffering from pain or for unknown causes of stomach discomfort.

Ingredients

1. 3 oz cut Peppermint leaves
2. 1 quart hot distilled water
3. 4 oz food grade vegetable glycerine

Method

1. Mix the Peppermint leaves in the hot distilled water.
2. Cover and let stand for 2 hours.
3. Bring the mixture to a boil then simmer gently for 5 minutes.
4. Add the glycerine and simmer for another 5 minutes.
5. Stain, cool and bottle the mixture.

Pest Deterrent

Peppermint can also be used as a pest deterrent. Ants and most other insects do not like the smell of peppermint. Mice and rats are also said to avoid peppermint although I have not found it to be an effective mouse deterrent.

Peppermint Cleaner

You can also use Peppermint to clean surfaces.

Ingredients

1. 1/2 c Peppermint
2. 1 quart water
3. 1/4 c distilled white vinegar
4. 10 drops tea tree oil (disinfectant)

Method

1. Steep the Peppermint in the water.
2. Remove the Peppermint and add the rest of the ingredients.
3. Mix and store the mixture in a spray bottle. Spritz to clean.

Food

According to the USDA, Peppermint is a good source of Vitamins A and C as well as minerals like Niacin, Phosphorus, Zinc, Riboflavin, Folate, Calcium, Iron, Magnesium, Potassium, Copper and Manganese. It is also a very good source of dietary fiber, making Peppermint a good addition to your diet.

The most common way to consume Peppermint is in tea form. Never boil the mint in water, which causes the volatile oils to evaporate and escape. Pour boiling water over your Peppermint leaves instead to retain the oils.

Cucumber, Chickpea Mint Salad

This recipe is best served the next day to allow the flavors to meld.

Ingredients

1. 1 cucumber, sliced
2. 1 cup of celery, sliced
3. 2 cups chickpeas, cooked and drained or one 15 oz can of chickpeas, drained
4. 3 medium-sized carrots, peeled and shredded
5. 1 cup fresh Peppermint, chopped
6. 1/4 cup raisins
7. 1 small white onion, peeled and sliced
8. 3 Tbsp red wine vinegar
9. 2 Tbsp extra virgin olive oil
10. 1 Tbsp honey (optional)
11. Salt and pepper to taste

Method

1. Toss the chickpeas, vegetables, Peppermint and raisins in a large bowl to mix.
2. In a small bowl, mix the vinegar, olive oil, honey and seasonings.
3. Drizzle the vinegar solution over the vegetables and toss gently to coat.
4. Cover the bowl and refrigerate overnight before serving.

- *Recipe adapted from allrooipos.com*

Peppermint Sauce

Mint sauce best accompanies roast lamb or fish.

Ingredients

1. 3/4 c finely chopped fresh Peppermint leaves
2. 2 tsp caster sugar
3. 1/4 c boiling water
4. 1/2 c white wine vinegar
5. A pinch of salt to taste

Method

1. Combine the mint and sugar in a heat-resistant bowl.
2. Pour the boiling water over the mixture and stir until the sugar dissolves.
3. Mix in the vinegar.
4. Add the salt.
5. Allow the sauce to stand for 15 minutes before serving.

- *Recipe adapted from taste.com.au*

Peppermint Vinegar

Mint vinegar goes well in fruit salads or accompanying lamb.

Ingredients

1. 2 c fresh Peppermint, washed, air-dried and chopped
2. 1 c white wine vinegar (it should be at least 5% acid, otherwise you'll run the risk of the infusion going bad)
3. 1-2 drops of green food coloring (optional)

Method

1. Add the Peppermint into a clean glass jar.
2. Pour the vinegar over the mint.
3. Add the coloring.
4. Cover tightly.
5. Allow the infusion to stand in a cool, dark place for 3 weeks.

Cultivation

Be careful where you plant Peppermint or any mint in general. It propagates easily and can become invasive. Peppermint spreads by runners and can quickly take over an area. If you have the space, plant it in an isolated area and let it spread.

If you have limited space, you can plant it in a barrel or fairly deep container sunk into the ground. Bear in mind that if your container is not tall enough (at least 14 inches), the mint runners can creep up from the drainage holes to invade your planting area. Some have also reported that planting Peppermint in a drier area helps to keep the plant growth in check.

Peppermint is a hardy perennial in Zones 5-9. I have, however, also been able to grow it with fair success as a perennial in Zone 4. It grows best in moist, rich loamy soil with good drainage, in full or partial sun. While Peppermint will grow in shady areas, it tends to get leggy. Planting in full sun also increases the potency of its oils and therefore the medicinal qualities of the Peppermint. Not enough sun and the plant gets leggy. It prefers slightly alkaline soils of pH 6.0-7.0. Keep your Peppermint bed well-watered and nutriented (dress with 2 inches of compost) every few weeks, especially if you harvest often.

Because Peppermint is a hybrid, its seeds will not grow true to its parent. It is therefore best to plant it from root or stem cuttings. Plant the Peppermint in spring, unless you have a frost-free climate in which case you can also plant in fall. Set the seedlings 18-24 inches apart or plant it in a pot that is at least 18 inches in diameter located in a sunny area.

You can prevent foliar diseases by having good air circulation between your plants. Keep the soil weed-free and consistently moist but not wet. Remove the flowers as they appear and cut the plant to the ground in fall. The Peppermint should return every year from the roots. Cover with a layer of straw mulch if your area suffers from long, hard frosts.

Harvesting

Keep cutting and harvesting the tops off your Peppermint when reaches about 12 inches tall to prevent it from getting leggy and to encourage bushy growth. Pick the larger outer leaves to encourage leaf growth.

Fresh leaves should be used immediately. You can also dry them by hanging the stems upside down in small bunches in a shaded area with good air circulation. The leaves are dry when they and the stems are brittle to the touch. Store the dried Peppermint in an airtight container.

Propagation

Divide your Peppermint plant every few years by digging up the plant in early spring before the plant starts sprouting. If needed, use a shovel or knife to cut the root ball apart and replant your divisions using the 18-24 inch plant spacing.

You can also propagate Peppermint from stem cuttings. To make a stem cutting, use a clean sharp knife to cut a leafy healthy peppermint stem (about 2 inches long). Pinch off the bottom leaves, leaving only the newest top leaves. Place your stem(s) in a shallow container of water, making sure that the leaf nodes that you stripped the leaves from are submerged in the water. The top leaves, however, should not touch the water surface.

Change the water every 3-4 days until the stem cutting starts to root. The rooting process may take over a month.

Transplant the cutting into a container of planting medium. Keep the potting medium consistently most but not wet. Covering the exposed soil and cutting in a clear plastic bag or dome with small vent holes can help to keep the moisture in. The new plant should be established in about 6 months.

Precautions

Although Peppermint use is generally safe, the University of Maryland Medical Center recommends taking any herb with caution, under the supervision of your healthcare provider because they can interact with other herbs, medications and/or supplements. Also consult your healthcare provider if you are pregnant or nursing.

Avoid taking Peppermint in any form if you suffer from GERD (gastroesophageal reflux disease) or hiatal hernia because Peppermint may relax the sphincter between the esophagus and stomach thereby worsening heartburn and indigestion symptoms. Peppermint may also make gallstones worse. Other possible interactions may include interactions with drugs that reduce stomach acids, treat diabetes or hypertension. Medications that are metabolized by the liver may also be affected by Peppermint.

Peppermint oil is the oil extract whereas a tincture is an infusion of peppermint in a carrier oil, which is not as concentrated as the oil extract or essence. Large doses of Peppermint oil can be toxic. Peppermint oil should also never be applied to a small child's or infant's face as it may cause spasms and inhibit breathing. The oil may also cause rashes when applied to the skin. Never use undiluted Peppermint oil internally. Ingesting as little as 1 teaspoon (2 grams) or menthol can be fatal.

8 RASPBERRY

Often used for its fruit production, red Raspberry also has wonderful curative properties. It is not surprising that the late famous British herbalist, Henry Box, declared that red Raspberry leaves are "the best gift god ever gave to women."

The red Raspberry (*Rubus idaeus; Rosaceae*) plant is a woody perennial that belongs to the rose family. It grows wild in many parts of the US, Canada, Japan, as well as parts of the UK. Cultivated variety are native to Europe and Asia.

Raspberry grows to heights of 5-8 feet, bearing large pinnate compound leaves, each with 5-7 leaflets which usually do not bear flowers. It starts producing side shoots and 0.5 inch, five-petalled white flowers in its second year. In summer to early fall, it produces edible sweet but tart fruit. Raspberries do not technically produce berries but rather, produce an aggregate fruit of numerous drupelets around a central core that separates from its core when picked.

Uses

Healing Agent

Red Raspberry leaf tea is not to be confused with the Raspberry fruit tea, where the fruit, rather than the leaves are infused in water. Raspberry leaf tea has a recorded history going as far back as the 1500s. It has been used in Europe, China, North and South America for centuries and has earned its place as the herb for pregnant or to-be-pregnant women.

During World War II, when drugs were hard to obtain in in England, researchers recommended that women consume the leaf tea to aid their pregnancy. Red Raspberry leaf tea is very high in important nutrients that are needed to support pregnancy including iron, calcium and Vitamins C and B. It also contains healing potassium compounds such as potassium chloride and potassium sulfate as well as calcium chloride, malic acid and other organic acids, all of which are necessary to promote tissue healing, which is important for mothers-to-be.

Moreover, Raspberry leaf tea also contains magnesium, potassium and iron which may help reduce nausea and leg cramps during pregnancy. According to Dr. Christopher, his colleague, Dr. Zofchak learned that red Raspberry leaf tea also helps to strengthen fetal attachment and its iron citrate content helps to ease the delivery process by helping the uterus contract more efficiently.

According to a study published in the 2001 Journal of Midwifery and Women's Health, women who drank Raspberry leaf tea had a shorter labor and fewer of their babies were delivered by forceps. Another study citing The Natural Pharmacist that was published in the Australian College of Midwives Journal, stated: "An unexpected finding in this study seems to indicate that women who ingest Raspberry leaf might be less likely to receive an artificial rupture of their membranes, or require a Cesarean section, forceps or vacuum birth than the women in the control group."

Of course, consume the tea in moderation. Dr. Christopher recommended consuming a cup of tea, three times a day during pregnancy to help to prevent nausea, first trimester spotting, and to help to increase the uterine wall muscle tone. After birth, the Raspberry leaf tea is said to help to reduce postpartum bleeding.

Some women even drink the tea during labor or suck on pre-frozen tea cubes, which supposedly helps to expel the placenta and encourage as well as enrich the mother's breast milk. Raspberry leaves contain pectin which has been found to be a soothing, healing agent. Drinking the tea after childbirth is believed to help to nourish the new mother and to restore the reproductive system.

If you do not like the flavor of Raspberry leaf tea, Dr. Christopher recommended consuming the berries freely, which offers similar effects of the leaf tea. The Raspberry fruits are also said to help to break up and to expel kidney and gall bladder stones.

Pest Deterrent

You can use Raspberry canes (or any other brambles) as a pest deterrent. Lay down the thorny canes gently over your young plants in a fairly dense mat. The Raspberry cane mat will still allow the plant to grow, receive light and water but the thorns will help to keep pests like deer away from the growing plant. It is a natural and free solution to a deer problem and I cannot recommend it enough for a prepper homestead.

Raspberry Muffins

Ingredients

1. 2 cups all-purpose flour
2. 1 1/4 cup sugar
3. 1 cup fresh Raspberries
4. 1/2 cup butter, melted
5. 3/4 cup milk
6. 2 eggs
7. 1/4 cup lemon juice
8. 1 Tbsp baking powder
9. 1/2 tsp salt
10. 1/2 tsp lemon zest (optional)

Method

1. Preheat oven to 400°F.
2. Line 12 muffin cups with paper muffin liners.
3. Combine all the dry ingredients except the Raspberries in a large bowl.
4. Sour the milk by mixing the lemon juice with the milk in a bowl.
5. Allow the mixture to rest for a few minutes.
6. Beat the eggs and stir the egg mixture into flour mixture until just moistened.
7. Fold in the Raspberries.
8. Fill the prepared muffin cups two-thirds full with the muffin batter.
9. Bake the muffins in the preheated oven for about 15 to 20 minutes or until a toothpick comes out clean when poked into a muffin.

10. Allow the muffins to cool for 5 minutes before removing the muffins from the pan to cool further.

- *Recipe adapted from AllRecipes.com*
-

<u>Raspberry Jam</u>

Makes 7-8 half-pint jars

Ingredients

1. 9 c crushed Raspberries
2. 6 c sugar

Method

1. Sterilize your canning jars without the lids screwed on in boiling water.
2. In a separate pot, combine the Raspberries and sugar.
3. Bring the mixture to a boil slowly, stirring occasionally until sugar dissolves.
4. Cook rapidly to, or almost to, gelling point, depending upon whether a firm or soft jam is desired.
5. As mixture thickens, stir frequently to prevent sticking.
6. Pour hot jam into hot jars, leaving 1/4 inch headspace.
7. Wipe jar rims and screw on the lids until they are finger-tight.
8. Process for 5 minutes in a boiling water canner.

NOTE: If seedless jam is preferred, crushed berries may be heated until soft and pressed through a sieve or food mill; then add sugar and proceed as above.

- *Recipe from 2015 OSU Extension Master Food Preserver Program*

Simple Raspberry Vinaigrette

Ingredients

1. 1 Tbsp Raspberry jam
2. 1/4 c white wine vinegar
3. 1/3 c extra virgin olive oil
4. Salt and black pepper to taste

Method

1. Whisk the first three ingredients together until well-mixed.
2. Season to taste.

Cultivation

Raspberries can not only be categorized by color but also by whether they are summer-bearing (common) or everbearing. Unlike everbearing strawberries that bear fruit throughout the summer, everbearing Raspberries produce an early-summer berries on the previous year's branches and another crop in fall on the current season's growth. Everbearers will only give you a fall harvest if you mow them to the ground in the fall. Summer bearers on the other hand, won't fruit if mown to the ground in the fall. A healthy Raspberry plant will remain productive for 10 or more years.

Depending on the variety, this hardy perennial will grow in Zones 2-8. It will grow in any soil type but prefers neutral to slightly acidic loamy soil and full sun. Although Raspberries can be started from seeds, it's best to start them from plant canes. It's also best to start them in fall although most people plant them in spring. If you live in a warmer climate, you can even plant them in late winter.

Prepare the soil with compost or well-aged manure two weeks before planting. Soak your Raspberry canes in water for 1-2 hours before planting and plant it in a hole that is slightly deeper and larger than the container that your plant came in. Some varieties may need to have a trellis or support in place, preferably before planting so as not to disturb maturing plants.

Plant the canes about 3 feet apart in rows about 8 feet apart. Fertilize them annually with a nitrogen-rich fertilizer like fish meal or alfalfa pellets before mulching them well (about 4 inches) to keep the weeds out and moisture in. Provide the Raspberry plants with about an inch of water a week. Expect the canes to only produce leaves in its first year; developing fruits in its second year and beyond.

While Raspberry plants are quite forgiving, it's best to prune them to keep the quality and production of fruits up. Canes die after 2 years so prune them off in fall, after the fruits mature. If you remove the pruned debris, the pruning process also helps to get rid of pests that may otherwise overwinter.

As the plant matures over the next few years, start thinning out some of the first-year canes. Keep the most vigorous and healthy canes and remove old canes around it to give it about a six-inch space. Getting rid of the less prolific canes provides more light and nutrients to the remaining canes, resulting in bigger berries and more disease-resistant plants.

Harvesting

Leaves

Some sources suggest harvesting the leaves before the plant starts flowering but generally, you can harvest the leaves at any time that there are green leaves large enough to use. Harvest your leaves on a clear day.

To encourage constant fresh growth, harvest small leaf batches throughout the season. I prefer to harvest fresh growth by randomly harvesting alternating leaf sets along the branch. Leave the green stems on the harvested leaves.

Harvest more than you think you'll need because the leaves will shrink during dehydration.

You can either dehydrate your leaves, together with the stems, in a dehydrator at 115-135°F, or air-dry them out of direct sunlight in a single layer between two clean kitchen towels. As long as the leaves are not piled thickly during the dehydrating process, some overlap is fine. If you live in a humid area, use a dehydrator over air-drying.

The leaves are dried when they are crisp to the touch but still green. They may also become whitish on the bottom. Gently crush the leaves to your desired tea-leaf size and remove any stems that are too thick to break apart, especially if you intend to use your leaves in tea bags. Store the dried leaves in glass containers in a cool, dry place out of direct sunlight.

Berries

Except for some everbearing varieties that produce berries in their first year. Raspberries will generally bear fruit in the early summer of their second year, ripening over a two-week time frame. Harvest the Raspberries on a clear day, when they are dry; every couple of days as they ripen. When ripe, the berries will leave the vine willingly. If you have to tug on them, they are not yet ripe.

If kept in the fridge, the berries will last for about 5 days. Freezing them will extend their life considerably. To freeze, lay them in a single layer on a tray or cookie sheet and place it in the freezer. Once frozen, you can remove the berries and store them in a ziplock bag, removing as much air as possible. A good way to extract the air is to insert a clean straw into the bag and sucking up as much air as you can before carefully removing the straw and sealing your bag shut. You can also turn the berries into Raspberry jam and can them.

Propagation

Look for new red Raspberry shoots at the base of the plant in early spring, after all danger of frost has passed. These are much lighter in color than the older canes. Using a sharp gardening spade, vertically sever any new 6-8 inch tall shoots from the mother plant. This method should divide the root systems below the soil line.

Remove the new shoots and replant them in a new growing area. The shoots should be planted at the same depth that it was growing before it was severed from the parent. Plant your shoots about 3-5 feet apart. Mulch the area to help to keep it weed-free. Water well and fertilize as you would the older plants.

Precautions

Red Raspberry leaf tea has been used for centuries with little cause for concern. However, a 1954 study using isolated fractions from *Rubus sp.* showed that some of these fractions caused uterine contractions.

If in doubt, consult your medical care professional before using, especially if pregnant, nursing or on other supplements and/or medications. Some people may be allergic to Raspberry.

9 SAGE

Sage (*Salvia officinalis; (Labiatae)*) is a hardy perennial plant in zones 5-8. In hotter climates, Sage does not fare as well and is usually grown as an annual. It is part of the Mint family of plants. Its name, *Salvia*, is believed to mean "I Save." It could also come from the Latin Salveo meaning, "I am well", or from *salvere* - "to be saved". In any case, these possible name derivations suggest the prowess of the humble Sage plant.

A Mediterranean native, Sage is now naturalized in many parts of the world. Varieties can vary in size, color and foliage pattern, with foliage colors ranging from grey-green to green to yellow and even tri-colored. Common Sage bears ovate, soft and hairy grey-green leaves about 1.5 to 2 inches long and according to the Arabic name, is likened to a camel's tongue. Sage blossoms sometime in August with whorls of purplish flowers.

The entire plant exudes a strong but warm-scent and is somewhat astringent in taste. It prefers to grow in sunny, well-draining soil.

Uses

Healing Agent

Sage can nearly be called a cure-all. Its antiseptic properties is often used to sooth coughs, colds and other throat problems. You can make a Sage gargle for mouth or throat ailments by steeping 1 tsp of dried Sage leaves that are collected before the plant flowers, in 1/2 cup water for 30 minutes. This gargle is said to also be useful in treating bleeding gums.

Avoid using aluminum when steeping the herbs because the chemicals in the herbs may react with aluminum. This infusion may be mixed with honey and lemon. Alternatively, you can also make a gargle by infusing an ounce of Sage leaves in half a pint of hot apple cider vinegar, diluted in another half a pint of cold water.

Sage also arrests secretions and has been used to stop hemorrhages. Applying a strong Sage tea to small wounds is said to stop bleeding and help to soothe and heal raw skin abrasions.

When consumed, Sage tea may also help to reduce a nervous headache and to calm a nervous system. It may also help to reduce excessive menstrual flow as well as help to contract the uterus after birth. However, it may also dry a mother's milk. Some nursing mothers consume it cold when it's time to wean the baby.

Dr. Christopher recommended that the mother should drink a cup of Sage tea before each meal until the milk weans. This use for Sage may be effective in both humans as well as animals. However, always consult your medical care provider or veterinarian respectively before administering Sage tea on yourself or on your animals.

When drunk, Sage tea may also relieve flatulence, constipation and loss of appetite. Sage tea can be so potent that in his book, Dr. Christopher mentioned that a cup of tea of Sage and Peppermint, drunk twice a day, cured one of his patients of a kidney infection.

The Queen of Hungary's Water

Although the exact origins of The Queen of Hungary's Water, or Hungary Water, is undetermined, it has been used as a fragrance and remedy in Europe since around the fourteenth century. According to herbalist Rosemary Gladstar, the gypsies had many uses for it including using it as a hair rinse, mouthwash, headache remedy, aftershave and footbath.

The following recipe is adapted from Ms Gladstar's recipe and may be re-adapted to your personal preference. It works as an astringent for all skin types and works as a hair rinse.

Ingredients

1. 6 parts Lemon Balm
2. 4 parts Chamomile
3. 4 parts Rose petals
4. 3 parts Comfrey leaf
5. 2 parts Peppermint leaves
6. 1 part Lemon peel
7. 1 part Rosemary
8. 1 part Sage
9. 1 part dried Elder flowers
10. Enough organic apple cider vinegar to cover the ingredients

Method

1. Place the herbs in a large-enough clean glass jar.
2. Fill the jar with enough apple cider vinegar such that the vinegar sits 1-2 inches above the herb level.
3. Cover and allow it to sit in a warm location, undisturbed for 2-3 weeks.
4. After the 2-3 weeks, strain the herbs out and re-bottle.

The infused vinegar will keep indefinitely and does not need to be refrigerated.

Teeth Cleaning

Sage leaves can also be to cleanse and whiten teeth as well as to strengthen the gums. You can either brush your teeth with fresh Sage leaves, or add dried powdered leaves to your regular toothpaste or baking soda alternative before brushing your teeth.

Mood Uplifter

Who can't use a little perk-me-up especially when times are tough? Sage has been used to alleviate mild depression. It is also used to improve memory and mental facility as evidenced by a number of placebo-controlled, double-blind studies as reported in "Advances in Nutrition: An International Review Journal."

Mosquito Repellent

Sage may also be used to make mosquito repellents, although I cannot personally attest to how effective it really is. A mosquito repellent spray is not difficult to make. In a glass jar, cover equal parts of dried sage, rosemary, lavender and mint with apple cider vinegar at room temperature. Cover and shake the infusion up daily for two weeks.

Strain the herbs out and re-bottle the vinegar into spray bottles. Keep the repellent refrigerated for up to two weeks.

Food

Of course, Sage is probably best known for its use in food. Sage pairs well with eggs (in an omelette), with chicken or lamb, with onions in a stuffing and with fruits like apples and pineapples. Fresh Sage leaves are also delicious in sandwiches.

You can also make a Sage butter which goes very well on pastas and fish.

Sage Butter

Ingredients

1. 1/2 c butter, room temperature
2. 8-10 fresh Sage leaves, julienned
3. 2 large garlic cloves, peeled and minced (optional)
4. 1/4 tsp salt

Method

1. Using a fork, mix all the ingredients together well.
2. Place the softened butter-mix onto a piece of plastic cling wrap.
3. In the cling wrap, shape the butter into a cylindrical form.
4. Refrigerate until the butter hardens.
5. Remove the clip wrap and slice the butter into discs before using.

- *Recipe adapted from food.com*

Tuscan Herb Salt

Instead of buying expensive season salts which often have questionable ingredients, you can make your own very simple and delicious herb salt which goes well on meat. The amounts listed in this recipe can be modified to taste.

Ingredients

1. 1 c coarse sea salt
2. 1/2 c fresh rosemary leaves, washed and dried
3. 3/4 c fresh sage leaves, washed and dried
4. 1 Tbsp garlic powder
5. 1 Tbsp ground black peppercorns

Combine all the ingredients and store it in the fridge.

Cultivation

Sage grows best in Zones 5-8. In hotter or colder climates, Sage can be potted or grown as an annual. As a Mediterranean native, Sage is very drought-tolerant but grows best in an area with soil at a pH of about 6.5-7, with good soil drainage and a lot of sunshine. If you have clay soil, amend it with sand and compost before planting your Sage plants. Sage plants also grow well in clay or terracotta pots, which allow the soil to dry out a little better than other less porous planters.

Sage plants are easy to start from seeds but can also be started from a small plant. Start seeds indoors about 6 weeks before the last frost. Plant the seeds about 1/8 inch deep and 24-30 inches apart. The seeds will germinate in about 10-21 days.

Since mildew can be a problem for Sage plants, it's best to plant seedlings at least 18-24 inches apart to ensure good air circulation. Water young Sage plants sparingly by misting the plant until the soil is moist, rather than drenching the plant.

When the plant is mature, water only the soil around the plant when the soil feels dry to the touch. You may not need to water the Sage in areas of higher rainfall. You may side dress with some compost once during the growing season but it is not absolutely necessary. In early spring, after the danger of frost has past but before there is much new growth, prune off the older, woodier stems. Prune off about a third of each mature stem.

Harvesting

In the first year, harvest the Sage leaves sparingly by picking leaves off as needed. After the first year, you can harvest by cutting whole stems off the plant. As with most other herbs, it's best to harvest around mid-summer, just before the flowers bloom. Do your final full harvest about two months before the first frost, which will allow any fresh growth to mature before the onset of winter.

Propagation

Sage plants start becoming leggy and woody after about 3-5 years and will need to be replaced. In addition to replacing the plants with new plants or seeds, you can also generate new Sage plants by layering or with cuttings.

To propagate from cuttings, cut a existing sage branch about 3 inches from the top. Remove any leaves from the lower end of the branch. Dip the cut-end in rooting hormone and place it in sterile soil. Place a plastic bag with small holes punched into it over the entire cutting and the top of the exposed soil. Allow about 4-6 weeks for the roots to form before replanting the Sage in another pot or in the garden.

Layering is an even easier way of propagating your Sage. To layer, bend one of the existing Sage branches and use a small piece or wire or even a small rock to pin it to the ground. Leave about 4 inches from the top above the ground and strip off any leaves that are touching the ground. Roots will start to form about 4 weeks after you pin the stem to the ground. At this point, you can cut the new rooted branch from its parent and transplant it carefully to its new location.

Precautions

Consuming excessive amounts of Sage may result in headaches and irritability in some people. There are some medical literature reports of lip and mouth lining inflammation caused by consuming Sage tea.

Sage contains large amounts of a toxic chemical, thujone, which may cause convulsions. However, heating Sage eliminates most of this chemical, resulting in minimal final risk. Some people may be allergic to Sage.

10 (STINGING) NETTLE

Nettle (*Urtica dioica;* (*Urticaceae*)) is a dioecious, herbaceous perennial plant although it may be evergreen in areas with mild winters. It is best known for its hollow stinging hairs or "trichomes" that grow on the leaves and stems. These trichomes act like hypodermic needles which inject histamine and other chemicals that produce a stinging sensation when it comes in contact with human or other animal skin.

A native of Europe, Asia and parts of Africa and North America, Nettle prefers growing in temperate, moist, shady areas with high annual rainfall. It normally grows to about 3-7 ft tall in the summer before dying down to the ground in winter. **Nettle can be invasive**, with rhizomes and stolons that spread widely. Their leaves are green and soft, with serrated edges that end in a tip. They grow to about 1-6 inches in length, on a wiry, green stem. The greenish or brownish flowers are small and numerous. Most species bear many stinging hairs.

Nettle has a long history of being used as food, medicine and fiber.

Uses

Healing Agent

Nettle, like dandelion greens, horsetail, oats, watercress and mustard greens, is an excellent source of calcium. Additionally, Nettle contains iron, zinc, manganese, potassium, magnesium and Vitamin A. In times of high stress or anxiety, you may want to add more calcium to your diet because it helps to ease irritability, nervousness, muscle cramping and spasms and insomnia.

Because Nettle is high in Vitamin C, it has been traditionally used to treat scurvy. It can also be used as a constituent in a tea to help to soothe teething babies and children undergoing growth spurts.

High Calcium Children's Tea

Ingredients

1. 3 parts Rose hips
2. 2 parts Lemon Balm
3. 2 parts Oat Straw
4. 1 part Nettle
5. 1 part Raspberry leaves
6. 1/2 part Cinnamon
7. 1/2 part Nutmeg
8. Maple syrup to taste (optional)

Method

1. Pour boiling water over the herbs and steep for 30-60 minutes.
2. Strain before serving.

- *Recipe adapted from Rosemary Gladstar's recipe*

Rosemary Gladstar's suggested dosage is:

- 2 tsp for children 2-4 years
- 1 Tbsp for children 4-7 years
- 2 Tbsp for children 7-11 years
- 1 c or 8 oz for adults

Nettle is approved by the German Commission E for internal and external use against inflammation. For its diuretic properties, it is approved for use to support the lower urinary tract. If consumed during pregnancy, it is said to increase and enrich the mother's milk. However, it may suppress a new mother's lactation if consumed post-partum. Regardless, it has been successfully used against post-partum hemorrhaging. It may also help to alleviate PMS and menopause symptoms, strengthen kidneys as well as to make a good scalp and hair tonic.

Anecdotally, I've found Nettle to be very effective in preventing hay fever. I normally take one about 1 Tbsp of dried Nettle leaves, steeped to make a 16 oz cup of Nettle tea daily about 2 months before allergy season. I stop taking the tea once allergy season starts. I've not suffered from hay fever since I started this regimen.

Historically, Nettle was also used to help to clear phlegm in the lungs and bronchial tubes. It was also used as an anti-asthmatic. Dr. Christopher reported that a Nettle tea was effective as an anti-asthmatic if taken 3-4 times a day over a long period of time. To make the tea, steep an ounce of equal parts of Nettle, Comfrey and Mullein in boiled water and strain before consuming.

Food

As a food, Nettle makes a delicious spinach substitute. Use only the young plants (harvest before the plants flower in late spring to early summer) because older plants tend to be more stringy even after cooking.

Be sure to cook Nettle well to minimize any irritation during consumption. Always wear gloves when harvesting or handling fresh or raw Nettles.

Nettle Egg Drop Soup

Ingredients

1. 6 c chicken stock or chicken bone broth
2. 3 eggs, beaten
3. 2 handfuls of Nettle leaves, chopped
4. 2 garlic cloves, peeled and minced
5. 1/2 c Shaoxing wine or dry Sherry (optional)
6. Soy sauce, salt, sesame oil to taste
7. Cilantro, sliced for garnish

Method

1. In a stockpot, bring your chicken stock or broth to a rolling boil.
2. Remove the stock from the heat.
3. Using a spoon, start swirling the stock.
4. Slowly pour the beaten eggs such that it ribbons into the hot stock.
5. Bring the stock to a boil again before lowering it to simmer.
6. Add the Nettles to the stock and cook until tender.
7. Add the seasonings to taste, adding the sesame oil last, away from heat.
8. Garnish with cilantro before serving (optional). Serve hot.

Nettle Lasagna

Ingredients

1. 1 lb sweet Italian sausage, casings removed
2. 1 medium white onion, diced
3. 5 c loose Nettle leaves
4. 2 c fresh or frozen peas
5. 3 Tbsp + 6 Tbsp unsalted butter
6. 1/2 c all-purpose flour
7. 4 1/2 c whole milk
8. 1 c Parmcsan cheese, finely grated
9. 2 cloves garlic, peeled and minced
10. Salt and pepper to taste
11. 12 no-boil lasagna noodles

Method

1. Preheat oven to 350°F.
2. In a large saucepan, cook the sausage and break up the pieces over medium high heat.
3. Cook until the meat is no longer pink.
4. Using a slotted spoon, transfer sausage to paper towel-lined plate.
5. Into same saucepan, add 3 Tbsp butter, then add the onions.
6. Sauté until just softened and slightly golden brown.
7. Add the Nettle leaves and sauté until wilted.
8. Remove from heat and set aside.

Making the Roux:

9. In a different saucepan, melt the rest of the butter over high heat.
10. Stir in flour and cook for 2 minutes.
11. Whisk in the milk.
12. Bring to a boil. Keep stirring.
13. Reduce heat.
14. Simmer for another minute.
15. Remove from heat.
16. Whisk in Parmesan cheese, garlic and seasonings.
17. Spread 1/4 cup of the roux in a 9-by-13-inch baking dish.
18. Layer with noodles, half the sausage, one third of the remaining roux, and another layer of noodles.
19. Top with sautéed Nettles and onions, half the remaining roux, the remaining sausage and another layer of noodles.
20. Finish off by topping with the remaining roux.
21. Cover the dish with aluminum foil.
22. Bake for ~28 minutes or until top is golden and bubbly.
23. Let stand 10 minutes.
24. Serve hot.

- *Recipe adapted from thebittenword.com*

Vegetarian Rennet

Nettle juice can even be used as a vegetarian substitute for animal rennet in cheese-making. Use about half the amount of dried Nettle leaves as a substitute for the fresh leaves.

Method

1. Wash 2lbs of fresh Nettle leaves under cool, clean water.
2. In a large pot, add the leaves and enough water to cover the leaves.
3. Bring the water to a light boil then reduce the heat to a simmer for 30 minutes.
4. Add a heaping tablespoon of sea salt and stir to dissolve.
5. Line a colander with a cheesecloth.
6. Drain the Nettle water through the colander and collect the drained liquid.
7. The drained liquid is the vegetarian rennet.

The Nettle rennet will keep for a few weeks if stored properly refrigerated and covered, away from sunlight.

To make your cheese, use 1 cup of Nettle rennet to 1 gallon of warm milk. Use slightly less salt than the cheese recipe calls for because of the salt content in the Nettle rennet. It can be used with any milk but the Nettle rennet may develop a bitter flavor over time (over 2 months). You can overcome this problem by consuming the cheese when it is younger.

Fodder

Nettles were sometimes cultivated as fodder in Sweden and Russia. It was also used as a replacement to regular cloth by the German military during the war. It is said to also help to heal digestive problems in horses as well as to improve a cow's milk production.

However, most livestock will avoid consuming fresh Nettle because of its sting. You have to cut the Nettle and allow it to wilt and dry to help to reduce the sting. Pigs are usually fed boiled Nettles. Dried, powdered Nettles mixed into poultry food are said to fatten the birds and increase egg-production. Nettle seeds are also used to fatten fowl. The Dutch and Egyptians even feed Nettle seeds to their animals, which produces a sleek coat.

Fertilizer

Much like Comfrey, Nettles can also be used in compost-making. Just add them to your compost pile to help with humus formation. You can also cover the Nettle in water and allow it to decompose for three weeks. Spraying on this Nettle compost-tea helps to strengthen plants and helps them to overcome drought stress.

Fiber

"When the nettle is young, its leaf forms an excellent vegetable; when it matures, it has filaments and fibres like hemp and flax. Nettle fabric is as good as canvas."
- *Les Misérables* by Victor Hugo

Nettle fiber is stronger than Flax but is harder to extract. It can be spun and woven into cloths and as recently as World War I, was used by Germany and Austria to make textiles.

I have not tried this myself but according to Jonsbushcraft.com, this is how you can extract fibers and make Nettle cord:

Wear gloves when you are processing your Nettle fiber.

- Choose the tallest Nettles. Both green and purple ones work but purple Nettle fibers tend to be stronger than the green ones.
- Only use fresh Nettles.
- Cut the Nettles off at the base.
- With one hand, hold the Nettle at the base, then run the other hand up the stem a few times until all the leaves and stings have been removed.
- Using your fingers, gently squeeze the entire hollow stems flat. You can also use a stick to lightly tap on the stems to flatten them.
- Using your finger nails, pry the stem open downwards.

- Separate the inner woody membrane from the outer side by bending and pulling the woody part away from the outer side.
- Discard the inner woody center.
- Separate the outer fiber lengthwise into about 4 pieces.
- The fibers will dry and shrink and will need to be rehydrated before making your cords.

To make your cords:

- Hold your fibers on one end so that the other ends remain uneven.
- Dampen the fibers by running moistened fingers down the length of the fibers.
- Holding the fibers on both ends, twist the ends in opposite directions.
- The fibers will kink naturally to form a small loop of an "eye" which will be the start of your cord.
- Hold the "eye" kink and keep the fibers slightly separate.
- Using your thumb and index finger, keep the tension on the fibers and use a rolling action down their entire length.
- If the fibers are too thin or need to be lengthened, pinch another fiber of similar thickness to the end of your earlier fiber piece and proceed with the process.
-

Dyes

As an interesting note, although I won't discuss the details because making dyes are not advantageous to a prepper, Nettle is also used to dye wool green in Russia. The roots, boiled with alum are also used to dye yarn yellow.

Cultivation

Nettle can be invasive and grows best in Zones 5-8 but will also grow in Zones up to 3-10. It prefers to grow where the land has been disturbed, in full sun to partial shade but will tolerate medium shade. It will grow in range of soil pHs: between 5.5 to 7.5 and prefers slightly moist soil. It will, however, tolerate fairly wet soil.

Always protect your skin when dealing with Nettle. Nettle is normally weedy so to help to control its growth and spread, cut the flowering heads off (usually in late summer) to curb seed production. Pull out any plants that you find growing outside the area where you want the Nettles to grow.

It would be a good idea to locate your Nettle patch in a low foot-traffic area, where unwitting people and animals will not get stung by them.

Harvesting

The first few weeks after the Nettles first shoot up (before they reach about a foot tall), is the best time to harvest them. Wearing gloves, harvest the tops of the Nettle up to the top two or three pairs of leaves. Collect your harvest in a paper bag. You can use plastic but it tends to make the harvests sweat more than I like. If you are harvesting Nettle in summer, only harvest the top pair of leaves, which will be the most tender. The other parts of the plant, including the stems are too fibrous.

Use kitchen tongs or wear gloves when you prepare your Nettles during the cooking process, including during the time that you are washing and transferring the Nettles into your cooking pot.

Propagation

Admittedly, not many people actually propagate Nettle on purpose. However, you can cultivate Nettles by rubbing the mature seed heads and releasing the seeds over the area where you want them to grow. Plant the seeds in spring.

Both the seeds and rhizomes will grow in most soils. To propagate them from rhizomes, take root divisions in fall, after the foliage has died back.

Precautions

"Nettle in, Dock out" - old British rhyme

Stinging Nettle can of course, sting! Reactions to the Nettle sting will range from a small one to a more significant local reaction. Folklore remedies for the sting include rubbing the affected area with Dock, Nettle juice or with herbs from the mint family, particularly Peppermint. You can also try washing the affected area with soap and water.

Consuming too much Nettle may deplete the body of potassium so you have to increase your potassium intake with other fresh vegetables. Consuming older leaves may cause a laxative effect. They also contain cystoliths which can be a kidney irritant.

Nettle is also a diuretic which may cause uterine contractions so pregnant women and nursing mothers should consult their medical provider before consuming it. Avoid giving Nettle to children under 2.

11 YARROW

Yarrow (*Achillea millefolium;* (*Asteraceae*)) is an erect, herbaceous perennial plant. It produces one to a few stems that grow between 0.6 to 3.5 feet in height. The almost feathery leaves grow spirally and evenly distributed along the stem, where the largest leaves are at the bottom to middle sections of the stem.

The disk flowers range from a white to pink and usually consist of 3-8 ovate rays of about 15 to 40 flowers. Yarrow resembles Wild Carrot as well as Poison Hemlock but has a strong, sweetish smell reminiscent of chrysanthemums rather than carrots (in the case of Wild Carrot) or bad-smelling mouse (in the case of Poison Hemlock).

Yarrow is also known as nosebleed wort and soldier's woundwort, hinting at Yarrow's healing properties. It has a long history of being used as medicine for thousands of years. More recently, in the last few hundred years, it has also been used as a food source.

Uses

Healing Agent

Fever, Cold and Flu Remedy

In addition to consuming onions and garlic, which are the best natural remedies for colds and flus, some also drink a few cups a day of Gypsy tea, made from an infusion of Peppermint, Yarrow and Elderflowers as a remedy.

For low-grade fevers (below 104°F), Yarrow tea is used to help to raise the body temperature naturally, opening pores and promoting perspiration. The perspiration helps to keep the fever in check.

Stress, Anxiety and Cramp Relief

Yarrow contains anti-spasmodics that helps to sooth muscles and the digestive tract. It also contains small amounts of thujone which gives its sedative properties that may be comparable to marijuana. Thujone is poisonous in large amounts but Yarrow does not contain enough to be harmful.

Traditionally, Yarrow tea drunk twice a day, may not only help to relieve stress and anxiety, but may also help to relieve menstrual cramps and to control excessive menstrual bleeding, to ease insomnia, nausea, sore throat, indigestion and heartburn.

Yarrow Tea

Ingredients

1. 1 tsp dried Yarrow
2. 1 c boiling water
3. Honey or other sweetener to taste (optional)

Method

1. Put the Yarrow into a non-plastic cup.
2. Pour boiling water into the cup.
3. Allow it to steep for about 10 minutes.
4. Sweeten it to taste.

Once cooled, a few drops of a strong infusion of this unsweetened tea into the ears, may help to ease earaches. The unsweetened tea has also been used by different Native American tribes as a hair rinse, to soothe skin irritations. It is also applied to chapped hands and sore nipples.

Rosemary Gladstar's Cramp-Relief Formula

Ingredients

1. 1 part Crampbark
2. 1 part Pennyroyal leaf
3. 1 part Yarrow
4. Peppermint leaf (for flavor, optional)

Method

1. In a small saucepan, cover the Crampbark with cold water.
2. Cover and heat the saucepan slowly to a simmer, for around 20-45 minutes.
3. Remove from heat and add the remaining herbs.
4. Cover and steep for 15-20 minutes.
5. Strain.

Drinking 1/4 to 1/2 cup of this infusion every 15 minutes may help menstrual cramps to subside.

Healing Poultices

Native Americans have used Yarrow as a healing poultice (the plant is pulverized and mixed with water) for many applications. Applied externally, it is used to cure headaches, itching, bruises, children's rashes, to reduce sores and swelling and to cure collar sores on horses. Yarrow was also chewed to ease toothache. Its leaves encourage clotting and was applied fresh to stem nosebleeds.

To make a more portable healing agent, you can make an ointment out of Yarrow by covering slightly wilted chopped Yarrow flower heads and leaves in olive oil. Allow the Yarrow to infuse the oil in sunlight for several days. Strain and press the remaining oil out well.

Gently heat the infused oil in a pan and add enough beeswax such that it will harden when cool. Pour the mixture carefully into a suitable clean container and allow it to cool and harden. The ointment can be used to ease eczema or dry skin.

Companion Plant

When grown as a companion plant in small numbers, Yarrow helps most vegetables and increases the aromatic qualities of herbs. As a dynamic accumulator of nutrients including Potassium, Phosphorus and Copper, Yarrow helps to draw these nutrients from the lower layers of the soil into the plant.

These nutrients then accumulate in the leaves that when fallen off, return back to the top layers of the soil, helping to fertilize the plants around it. This process helps to improve the quality, rather than the quantity of the surrounding plants.

Fertilizer & Foliar Spray

Because it is a dynamic accumulator, Yarrow can also be used much like Comfrey, as a fertilizer and as a liquid plant feed. You can add Yarrow to your compost pile, or make a compost tea by soaking leaves in water for a few weeks, much like when making a Comfrey compost tea. Dilute 1 part compost tea in 20 parts water to make a foliar spray.

Beneficial Insect Attractant

Yarrow is a nectar plant and will attract beneficial insects, especially bees. It also provides shelter to a host of other beneficial insects including lacewings, beetles and spiders. As an additional advantage, Yarrow is also an aromatic pest confuser. That is, it is so strongly scented that it confuses pests and prevents them from finding vulnerable plants.

Food

Yarrow leaves can be used as a hops substitute for flavoring and as a preservative for beer-making. They are also edible and can be consumed raw or cooked but are bitter. It's best to consume the leaves young and mixed with other greens in a salad. However, some people may be allergic to Yarrow and it should not be consumed regularly.

Yarrow Omelette

Ingredients

1. 6 eggs, beaten
2. 1/4 c Yarrow, finely chopped
3. 1 small onion, finely chopped
4. 1-2 cloves of garlic, peeled and minced
5. 1 Tbsp butter or your cooking oil of choice
6. Salt and pepper to taste

Method

1. In a warm pan, melt your butter.
2. Add the onions and garlic and saute until tender.
3. Remove the onions and garlic to a separate bowl.
4. Reheat the pan and add more butter if needed.
5. Add the beaten eggs to the pan and cook until the eggs form a golden crust.
6. Add yarrow, onions and garlic to the eggs.
7. Add the salt and pepper to taste.
8. Fold the omelette over.
9. Cook until the eggs are firm.
10. Serve hot.

Cultivation

Yarrow is very forgiving in the garden and will grow even when trampled on. It does not need much space and will grow even in narrow beds. It is happiest in Zones 3-9 in full sun with dry to medium soil but will grow in a range of soil types from normal to sandy to clay, and in neutral, alkaline and acidic soils.

Its soil preference though, is well-drained sandy loam. It tolerates hot, humid weather and drought but does not like wet feet or moist, rich soil, which tends to make the plant flop. If kept unchecked, **Yarrow can be invasive** and may take over the area, spreading by roots as well as by seed.

Yarrow is usually propagated by division but can also be grown from seed. If planting from seed, the seeds need to first be stratified for about a month before the last frost date. Stratification tricks the seed into thinking that it is undergoing a winter.

To stratify the seeds, wet a paper towel and squeeze any excess water out. Lay the wet paper towel flat and space out the Yarrow seeds on one side of the paper towel. Fold the paper towel over and place it in a ziplock bag. Seal and refrigerate. Leave it undisturbed for a month.

When planting your seeds, cover the seeds about 1/4 inch deep, in moist potting soil and place the pots in a sunny, warm area. You can cover the top of the pot with a plastic bag or plastic wrap with small air holes. The seeds should germinate in about a week. Remove the plastic as soon as the seeds sprout. Space your seedlings about 1-2 feet apart, in loosened soil mixed with about 1 inch of compost.

Plant Yarrow cuttings in spring or summer. Water regularly if you get less than 1 inch of rain per week in summer. Mulch around your plants, adding about 2 inches of mulch and a thin layer of compost (optional) each spring. To help to keep your Yarrow bushy, cut back some of the plant stems in late spring, before they start flowering. Divide clumps in spring every 2-3 years to keep the parent plant healthy.

Harvesting

Harvest Yarrow after it has started flowering, by collecting the entire plant. Choose a warm, sunny day to harvest, after the dew has dried but before it gets hot enough to cause the essential oils to dissipate.

Collect the flower heads by cutting the flowers away from the stem and collecting them. Running your fingers down the stem strips the leaves off easily. If the plant has off-shoot branches, cut those off before running your fingers down the primary stem.

Propagation

Yarrow is best propagated by stem cuttings collected between late spring and summer. Using clean pruning shears, quickly and evenly take about 6-inch long cuttings that have about 3-4 buds from new and healthy stems. Take cuttings near or just below the soil line.

Place your cuttings in a small pot of good-draining potting mix. The potted cuttings should be in a sunny and warm place (the University of Maryland recommends keeping the temperature at between 50-60°F). Once the stems form roots about 1 inch in length, you can transplant them in a sunny area outside. You can also directly plant any Yarrow divisions in new sunny locations.

To plant from seed, collect seeds from brown, faded blooms on a clear day. The stems should be dried at least 6 inches from the flower head and should appear dark brown or black. Cut the stem and seed head off and place it in a paper bag.

To collect the seeds, place a newspaper sheet under the flower head. Hold the stem and turn the flower head upside-down. Gently tap the dried flower or use the palm of your opposite hand to gently squeeze the flowers to release the seeds. Both the tiny seeds and chaff will be released. Do not worry about removing the chaff -- it will take care of itself when it is planted. Plant the seeds outdoors in a well-draining sunny location.

You can also propagate Yarrow by taking basal cuttings in spring. Unlike seed propagation, Yarrow plants propagated by basal cuttings may not bloom the first year. You can also divide plants after they have flowered in spring. Dividing plants every three to four years helps them to maintain heartiness. If starting seeds indoors to transplant later, start them about eight weeks before time to plant them outdoors in early spring.

Precautions

Yarrow is generally safe to use externally but some people may have allergic reactions like rashes or other unexpected side effects. Reduce the dosage or stop using if these occur and consult your medical provider if symptoms persist. High doses of Yarrow may also cause urine to turn dark brown. This is a harmless effect.

12 CONCLUSION

I hope that this book has provided you with a good start to planting a prepper or homestead medicinal garden. As you gain more confidence, look into adding more medicinal plants that suit to your region.

There are also many useful herbs and spices such as cinnamon, ginger and turmeric, which cannot easily be grown in North America. Even though they are not included in this book, these more tropical medicinal herbs and spices should have a place in your homestead or prepper pantry. To natural remedies and good health!

Sign up for new book release updates and FREE bonus e-book downloads at http://byjillb.com

ABOUT THE AUTHOR

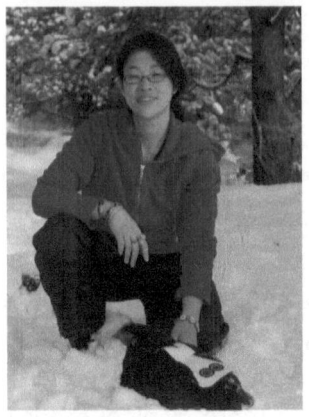

HomeGrown • HomeMade • HomeBusiness • HOMESTEAD

Jill Bong writes under the pen name Jill b. She is an author, entrepreneur, homesteader and is the co-inventor and co-founder of Chicken Armor (http://chickenarmor.com), an affordable, low maintenance chicken saddle. She has also written over a dozen homesteading and home business books.

With a no-nonsense style, Jill draws from her own experiences and mistakes, and writes books focusing on maximizing output with minimal input to save you time and money.

Jill has been mentioned/quoted in various publications including The Associated Press, The New York Times, The Denver Post and ABC News. She has written for various magazines including Countryside and Small Stock Journal, Molly Green, Farm Show Magazine and Backyard Poultry Magazine. She holds an Engineering degree from an Ivy League from a previous life.

At its height, her homestead included over 100 chickens, geese and ducks, as well as cats, a dog, bees and a donkey named Elvis. She currently lives on her homestead in rural Oregon.

Learn more by visiting her site http://byjillb.com.

Books By Jill b.

Please check out my other books at **http://byjillb.com**:

The Modern Frugal American Housewife Book #1
Home Economics

The Modern Frugal American Housewife Book #2
Organic Gardening

The Modern Frugal American Housewife Book #3
Moms Edition

The Modern Frugal American Housewife Book #4
Emergency Prepping

CAN Dos and Don'ts
Water Bath and Pressure Canning

How to Keep Backyard Chickens
A Straightforward Beginner's Guide

The Best Backyard Chicken Breeds
A List of Top Birds for Pets, Eggs and Meat

Foraging
A Beginner's Guide to Wild Edible and Medicinal Plants

Medicinal Herb Gardening
10 Plants for The Self-Reliant Homestead Prepper

How to Make Money on eBay: Beginner's Guide

From Setting Up Accounts to Selling Like a Pro

How to Make Money on eBay: Maximize Profits

Secrets, Stories, Tips and Hacks - Confessions of a 16-Year eBay Veteran

How to Make Money on eBay: International Sales

Taking the Fear and Guesswork Out of Doing Business Internationally on eBay

Self-Publishing on a Budget with Amazon

A Guide for the Author Publishing eBooks on Kindle

DISCLAIMER & DISCLOSURE

This book does not contain medical advice. The contents of this book are for educational and informational purposes only. While many plants may have healing properties, the statements and/or uses have not been approved by the FDA. None of the information should be construed as medical advice nor should it be used as a substitute or replacement for conventional medicine, prescription drugs or medical care by a trained medical professional.

Ingesting herbs can interact with medications and interfere with their effectiveness or cause an adverse reaction to occur. Even though there are historical anecdotes of how some herbs have helped with life-threatening conditions, no herbal remedy should be administered without the supervision of a medical professional. Always consult a medical doctor before using any herbal remedies.

This guide is for entertainment and informational purposes only. The author and anyone associated with this book shall not be held liable for damages incurred through the use of information provided herein. Content included in this book is not intended to be, nor does it constitute, the giving of financial, legal or professional advice.

The author and others associated with this book make no representation as to the accuracy, completeness or validity of any information in this book. While every caution has been taken to provide the most accurate information, please use your own discretion before making any decisions based solely on the content herein. The author and others associated with this book are not liable for any errors or omissions nor will provide any form of compensation if you suffer an inconvenience, loss or damages of any kind because of, or by making use of, the information contained herein. Any opinion given is the author's own, based on her experience. If in doubt, always seek the advice of a professional who can advise you appropriately before acting on any part of this book.

This book contains references and links to other Third Party products and services. Some of these references have been included for the convenience of the readers and to make the book more complete. They should not be construed as endorsements from, or of any of these Third Parties or their products or services. These links and references may contain products and opinions expressed by their respective owners. The author does not assume liability or responsibility for any Third Party material or opinions. Links denoted by an asterisk (*) may contain affiliate links for which the author may receive compensation for click-through purchases.

BIBLIOGRAPHY

Almanac.com

Babycentre.co.uk

BHG.com

Bonnieplants.com

Canadiangardening.com

Culturesforhealth.com

Garden.org

Gardensablaze.com

GardenGuides.com

Gardeningknowhow.com

Herbs2000.com

Herb Syllabus Master Herbalist Guide, Dr. John R. Christopher (Christopher Publications, 2010)

Heirloom-Organics.com

Jonsbushcraft.com

LiveStrong.com

MedicinalHerbInfo.org

Missouribotanicalgarden.org

Motherandchildhealth.com

Motherearthliving.com

Mother Earth News Magazine

NourishedKitchen.com

Plants for a Future

Rosemary Gladstar's Family Herbal: A Guide to Living Life with Energy, Health, and Vitality , Rosemary Gladstar (Storey, 2001)

Seeds from Italy

Tcpermaculture.blogspot.com

TheGardenHelper.com

The New Healing Herbs, Michael Castleman (Rodale, Inc, 2009)

USDA NRCS Plant Guide

University of Maryland Medical Center

Wikipedia.org

Cover image credit: Raspberry © Bjørn Hovdal | Dreamstime.com